D1103944

Discourse, the Body, and Identity

Discourse, the Body, and Identity

Edited by

Justine Coupland and Richard Gwyn

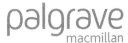

First published 2003 by
PALGRAVE MACMILLAN
Houndmills, Basingstoke, Hampshire RG21 6XS and
175 Fifth Avenue, New York, N. Y. 10010
Companies and representatives throughout the world

PALGRAVE MACMILLAN is the global academic imprint of the Palgrave
Macmillan division of St. Martin's Press, LLC and of Palgrave Macmillan Ltd.
Macmillan® is a registered trademark in the United States, United Kingdom
and other countries. Palgrave is a registered trademark in the European
Union and other countries.

ISBN 0–333–96900–6

This book is printed on paper suitable for recycling and made from fully
managed and sustained forest sources.

A catalogue record for this book is available from the British Library.

Library of Congress Cataloging-in-Publication Data
Discourse, the body, and identity/edited by Justine Coupland and
Richard Gwyn.
    p. cm.
Includes bibliographical references and index.
ISBN 0–333–96900–6 (cloth)
   1. Body, Human–Social aspects. 2. Sociolinguistics. 3. Body language.
4. Identity (Psychology) I. Coupland, Justine. II. Gwyn, Richard, PhD.
HM636 .D57 2002
306.4–dc21   2002073711

10   9   8   7   6   5   4   3   2   1
12   11   10   09   08   07   06   05   04   03

Printed and bound in Great Britain by
Antony Rowe Ltd, Chippenham and Eastbourne

Contents

Part 3   The Body, Pathology and Constructions of Selfhood

Editors' Preface and Acknowledgements

This book grew from one of a series of meetings of the Cardiff Roundtable in Language and Communication, all of which have been held at the University of Wales conference centre at Gregynog Hall (Newtown, Mid-Wales). The Roundtable on the theme 'Discourses of the Body' was held in June 1999. This was the fourth Roundtable. The themes of the first three were 'Approaches to Media Discourse', 'Sociolinguistics and Social Theory' and 'The Sociolinguistics of Metalanguage'. These have all in turn led to edited volumes. A fifth meeting, in 2001, was held on the theme of 'Narrative as a Resource' and a sixth, in 2002, on 'Language and Global Communication'. The Roundtable series is designed as a way of integrating and critically assessing research themes that have particular salience in sociolinguistics, discourse, or the study of human communication generally. Each Roundtable works by bringing together researchers who have distinctive personal or disciplinary perspectives on the designated theme and substantial research experience to draw on. The meetings at Gregynog Hall allow the privilege of physical, social and intellectual space for intensive discussion, debate and development of the relevant themes.

Like the other books emanating from the Roundtables, *Discourse, the Body and Identity* is not a proceedings volume. Not all the contributors to the Roundtable were able to contribute, and two of the chapters, by Kathleen Woodward and by Deborah Lupton and Wendy Seymour respectively, have been added to the set emerging from the original meeting. The chapters are the result of significant reworking of the original papers presented. The time that has elapsed between the Roundtable and the publication of this volume has been longer than we originally intended. As editors, we are grateful to our contributors for their patience, which we take as reflecting their faith in the project, and we have no doubt that a more stimulating collection has emerged as a result of the additional time we have all been able to give our contributions and we (as editors) have been able to give to our overseeing of them.

'The Body' is currently the focus of concerted and energetic interest across a wide range of academic disciplines. This book brings a wide range of these disciplines together in one volume, integrating contributions from authors well known for their work in sociolinguistics, conversation analysis and ethnomethodology, discursive psychology, sociology, and cultural and critical communication studies. Taken together, the chapters provide much-needed grounded analyses of texts on the body, talk about the body and embodied interaction, produced from this range of interdisciplinary perspectives.

We are grateful to the British Academy for financial support for the Roundtable on 'Discourses of the Body', alongside support given by the Centre for Language and Communication Research, Cardiff University. Particular acknowledgement is due to our colleague Adam Jaworski, who played at least an equal role to the two editors in the organisation and stewardship of the Roundtable, and in the early stages of the planning and preparation of this volume. Without his contributions, the book would not have existed in its current form. We would also like to thank Charles Goodwin for the insight and inspiration provided to the editors by his commentaries during the Roundtable itself. Finally, Nik Coupland deserves a great deal of recognition for his unfailing encouragement and intellectual support.

References

Bell, A. and Garrett, P. (eds) (1998) *Approaches to Media Discourse*. Oxford: Blackwell.

Coates, J. and Thornborrow, J. (eds) (in preparation) *The Sociolinguistics of Narrative*.

Coupland, N. Sarangi, S. and Candlin, C. (eds) (2001) *Sociolinguistics and Social Theory*. London: Longman/Pearson Education.

Jaworski, A., Coupland, N. and Galasinski, D. (in press) *The Sociolinguistics of Metalanguage*. Berlin: Mouton de Gruyter.

Notes on the Contributors

Justine Coupland is Senior lecturer at the Centre for Language and Communication Research at Cardiff University. She has published widely on discourse and identity, communication and the lifespan and conversational ritual in journals including *Language in Society, Discourse and Society, Text, Journal of Pragmatics, Journal of Sociolinguistics* and *Research on Language and Social Interaction*. Her publications include *Small Talk* (2000), the *Handbook of Communication and Aging Research* (1995, with Jon Nussbaum), *Language, Society and the Elderly* (1991, with Nikolas Coupland and Howard Giles), and *Contexts of Accommodation* (1991).

Charles Goodwin is Professor of Applied Linguistics at the University of California at Los Angeles. Publications include *Conversational Organization: Interaction Between Speakers and Hearers* (1977), *Rethinking Context: Language as an Interactive Phenomenon* (edited with Alessandro Duranti, 1992), *Conversation and Brain Damage* (editor, 2002) and numerous book chapters and articles in journals including *American Anthropologist, Research on Language in Social Interaction, Social Studies of Science, Mind, Culture and Activity* and the *Journal of Pragmatics*. His interests include study of the discursive practices used by hearers and speakers to construct utterances, stories and other forms of talk, language in the professions, the ethnography of science, cognition in the workplace and aphasia in discourse.

Richard Gwyn is Senior Lecturer in the School of English, Communication and Philosophy at Cardiff University. His research interests include autobiographical narratives, the cultural mythology of illness and media representations of the body. He has been involved in joint research with colleagues at the University of Wales College of Medicine into shared decision-making in general practice, and is currently lead researcher in a study of patient narratives of chronic fatigue. He is the author of *Communicating Health and Illness* (2002).

Christian Heath is a Professor in the Management Centre, King's College, London, and Director of the Work, Interaction and Technology Research Group. He holds visiting Professorships at the

Universities of Konstanz, Paris and Lyon and is a member of various editorial boards and co-editor of the series *Learning and Doing*. His publications include seven books, various television and in-house programmes and more than one hundred articles in academic journals and books. Recent and forthcoming publications include articles in the *British Journal of Sociology, Sociology* and *Mind, Culture and Activity*. He is also co-author of *Technology in Action* and co-editor of *Workplace Studies* (2000).

Mike Hepworth is Reader in Sociology at the University of Aberdeen and Visiting Professor of Sociology at the University of Abertay Dundee. He is also a Past By Fellow of Churchill College, Cambridge. Originally a sociologist of crime and deviance, his main research interests are in the sociology of the body and the sociology of ageing. The specific focus of his research is on the role of visual and verbal images in the social construction of ageing. He has published widely in this area and his latest book, a study of representations on ageing in popular fiction, is *Stories of Ageing*. He is currently working on images of ageing in Victorian painting. He is a founder member of the journal, *Theory, Culture and Society*, and member of the editorial board of the journal *Body & Society*. His professional associations include membership of Age Concern Scotland, the British Society for Social Gerontology, and the British Sociological Association.

Jon Hindmarsh is a Research Fellow of the Work, Interaction and Technology Research Group in the Management Centre, King's College, London. His principal area of research interest is the interactional organisation of talk and embodied conduct, particularly within workplace settings. Recent or forthcoming publications include articles in *Sociology, the Journal of Pragmatics*, the *Journal of Contemporary Ethnography* and the *Sociological Quarterly*. He is also co-editor of *Workplace Studies* (2000).

Adam Jaworski is Reader at the Centre for Language and Communication Research, Cardiff University. His book publications include *The Power of Silence: Social and Pragmatic Perspectives* (1993), *Silence: Interdisciplinary Perspectives* (1997), *Sociolinguistics: A Reader and Coursebook* (with Nikolas Coupland, 1997) and *The Discourse Reader* (with Nikolas Coupland, 1999). He is involved in two research projects, funded by The Leverhulme Trust, on reporting the future in radio news broadcasts, and language and tourism as a global cultural industry.

Deborah Lupton is Professor of Sociology and Cultural Studies at Charles Sturt University, Australia. She is the author/co-author of eleven books and editor of another, the most recent of which include *The Emotional Self: A Sociocultural Exploration* (1998), *Risk* (1999), *Risk and Sociocultural Theory: New Directions and Perspectives* (1999) and *Risk and Everyday Life* (2003). Her current research interests include the sociocultural aspects of risk; the body; technoculture; medicine and public health; and parenthood.

Ulrike Hanna Meinhof is Professor of German and Cultural Studies in the School of Modern Languages at the University of Southampton. Her current work on identity construction focuses on three generation families in European border communities (2000–3), and a new project investigates cultural policy in European cities in relation to people from ethnic minorities (2002–5). In both of these areas she is co-ordinating and conducting research financed by the European Commission's Fifth Framework programme. Recent publications include: *Living (with) Borders: Identity Discourses on East–West Borders in Europe* (2002) *Intertextuality and the Media: From Genre to Everyday Life* (2000, with J. Smith, eds), *Worlds in Common? Television Discourse in a Changing Europe* (1999, with Kay Richardson), *Language Learning in the Age of Satellite Television* (1998), *Masculinity and Language* (1997, with S. Johnson, eds).

Alan Radley is Professor of Social Psychology in the Department of Social Sciences at Loughborough University. He is the editor of *Health: An International Journal for the Social Study of Health, Illness and Medicine*. His research interests include the social context of health and illness and, more recently, questions of visual representation. He has written about the body in these contexts as well as with reference to the material world. His book publications include *Prospects of Heart Surgery: Psychological Adjustment to Coronary Bypass Grafting* (1988); *The Body and Social Psychology* (1991); *In Social Relationships: An Introduction to the Social Psychology of Membership and Intimacy* (1991); *Making Sense of Illness: The Social Psychology of Health and Disease* (1994). He is editor of *Worlds of Illness: Biographical and Cultural Perspectives on Health and Disease* (1993).

Wendy Seymour is an Adjunct Associate Professor at the University of South Australia. Her research interests are centred on computer communication technologies, disability, gender, the body and research methodologies. Her publications include *Remaking the Body: Rehabilitation and Change* (1998). She has published numerous chapters and journal articles on the body, health, and physical disability in *Qualitative Research, Journal of Australian Studies,* the *Journal of Occupational Science* and *Social Science and Medicine.*

John Tulloch is Professor of Media Communication at Cardiff University and Director of the Centre for Cultural Research (CCRR) into Risk at Charles Sturt University. He was the lead researcher (with Deborah Lupton) of a major Fear of Crime report in Australia, and while at Cardiff has written and published on television audience research, performance and culture, and several articles on perceptions of risk with Deborah Lupton. He is currently completing books on theories and methods of live audience analysis, and *Risk and the Everyday* (with Deborah Lupton).

Marian Tulloch is a Senior Lecturer in Psychology and Head of the School of Social Sciences and Liberal Studies at Charles Sturt University, New South Wales, Australia. She has researched and published in a range of areas relating to television, gender, violence and crime with a particular interest in the combining of quantitative and qualitative research methodologies. She was part of an interdisciplinary team from the Centre for Cultural Research into Risk, which conducted a national consultancy into fear of crime in Australia.

Kathleen Woodward is Professor of English at the University of Washington, where she directs the Simpson Center for the Humanities. The author of *Aging and Its Discontents: Freud and Other Fictions* (1991) and the editor of *Figuring Age: Women, Bodies, Generations* (1999) and *The Myths of Information: Technology and Postindustrial Culture* (1980), she is working on a book entitled *Circulating Anger and Other Feelings: The Cultural Politics of the Emotions.* Her essays have appeared in *Substance, Discourse, American Literary History, Cultural Critique, and Generations* as well as in collections of essays, including *Freud and the Passions* (1996), *Images of Ageing: Cultural Representations of Later Life* (1995), and *Culture on the Brink: Ideologies of Technology* (1994). She is the Chair of the National Advisory Board of Imagining America, an organization devoted to the arts and humanities in public life.

1
Introduction

Justine Coupland and Richard Gwyn

Social science discovered 'embodiment' late in the twentieth century. This was part of a significant theoretical shift, with developments in critical and cultural theory making 'discourse' available as an explanatory concept. At its most general, the argument was that social and cultural life is invested with meaning and value by regular symbolic representations. Discourse, in Foucault's sense, could be seen to act as a predisposing mechanism and as a social filter for possible meaning. The perspective breathed new life into social analysis, which was trapped in several dualistic assumptions. One of these was that cognitive and behavioural dimensions of experience should be radically separated. Linguistics was similarly compartmentalised, with the effect that meaning was either ignored or sequestered into narrow aspects of analysis (mainly lexical). Another was the structure – agency dualism, where a presupposed structural model of social life seemed to leave little scope for human agency at all. In line with this, social processes, and particularly processes of meaning-making, seemed to have little relevance to social order. Steady growth in the scope and confidence of proponents of discourse analysis has led to a position where linguists, too, can play a part in social analysis – and not merely as empiricists testing out the social theories of social scientists. In fact their role now is arguably a central one, offering more systematic theoretical-plus-empirical orientations to social meaning and social practice. In just this spirit, the present volume offers a series of detailed, empirically grounded studies of discourses of the body.

Behind this enterprise the presence of two key figures looms large. Were it not for the work of Erving Goffman and Michel Foucault, social scientific perspectives on the body would be radically different. For Goffman (1959), individuals are ceaselessly staging performances

1

whose aim is to enhance their own interests and minimise loss of face. Central to this notion of the presentation of self is the maintenance of a positive and convincing self-image. Modern societies have gradually put in place many criteria for an ideal body-image, manifested most openly in the idea of the commodified body, and supported by industries that provide specifically for body-care, dieting and keeping fit. Goffman's discussion of the body is motivated by three principal ideas:

1. the body is the material property of individuals, which individuals control and monitor in order to interact;
2. individuals present and manage their bodies in accordance with shared vocabularies of body-idiom that are not individually controlled but hierarchically set and symbolically charged;
3. the body mediates the relationship between self-identity and social identity: consequently, the social meanings attached to bodily display and expression are an extremely important factor in an individual's sense of self, and his or her feelings of inner worth (cf. Shilling, 1993: 82–3).

Goffman's work relates principally to the healthy body, and the ways in which people devise and maintain strategies for successfully managing interactions with each other. In particular he is concerned with the presentation of self, and the remarkable competence that individuals show in managing the expressions, movements and gestures involved in communicative interactions. According to Goffman, both face work (the maintenance of positive 'face' in social interaction) and body work ('body language', gesture and eye contact, proxemics and touch) are crucial to the successful negotiation of encounters and the establishing and maintaining of social roles.

Of particular interest to us is the way that Goffman (in *Stigma*, 1968) examines the problems of the disabled, and the chronically disfigured, not only because of the extra work such people need to do in order to be fully included as members of society, but also because any study of the disabled brings into sharp focus the divergence between individuals' 'virtual social identity' and their 'actual' social identity, that is, the ways in which they believe themselves to be perceived by an other as opposed to the ways in which they are perceived in actual practice. This ambivalence of perception, between the virtual and the actual, finds its correspondence in the unspoken dialogue that underpins all relations between the self and the imagined other, invoking a pervasive self-examination and attention to appearance.

The debt to Foucault in almost any enterprise concerned with the discourse of the body in contemporary social science cannot be understated. For Foucault, and for the many scholars he has influenced, the body is 'the ultimate site of political and ideological control, surveillance and regulation' (Lupton, 1994: 23). Since the eighteenth century, claims Foucault, the body has been subjected to a unique disciplinary power. It is through controls over the body and body behaviours that state apparatuses such as medicine, schools, psychiatry and the law have been able to define and delimit individuals' activities, punishing those who violate the established boundaries and maintaining the productivity and political usefulness of bodies.

The Foucauldian approach to the body is characterised, first, by a substantive preoccupation with those institutions that govern the body and, second, by an epistemological view of the body as produced by and existing in discourse. Bodies that were once controlled by direct repression are, in high modernity, controlled by stimulation. Thus the body in consumer culture is coerced into a normative discourse ('Get undressed – but be slim, good-looking, tanned', as Foucault reminds us). Bodies for Foucault are 'highly malleable phenomena which can be invested with various and changing forms of power' (Shilling, 1993: 79).

Significantly, the body is under a dual scrutiny, observed both by others and with its 'own' eyes. It is the former that, in its most extreme and dispassionate sense, constitutes the 'clinical gaze', which Foucault defines as:

> a perceptual act sustained by a logic of operations; it is analytic because it restores the genesis of composition; but it is pure of all intervention insofar as this genesis is only the syntax of the language spoken by things themselves in an original silence. The gaze of observation and the things it perceives communicate through the same Logos, which, in the latter, is a genesis of totalities and, in the former, a logic of operations. (1973: 109).

The clinical gaze, the symbolic enactment of a corresponding 'medicalization' of society (*cf.* Illich, 1976), is, however, no longer the strict preserve of medical practitioners. With the evolution of an increasingly omnipresent visual culture and an abundance of films and television documentaries concerned with issues of the body, illness and human decrement, we are all, to an extent, invited to be witnesses, to share in the clinical gaze as participant observers in a mass-mediated ethno-

graphic exercise. Voyeurs all, we necessarily turn our gaze upon ourselves, and it is this introspection that informs a perpetual striving to
meet an ideal configuration of body and selfhood, which might
express itself in countless ways, but each dedicated to rooting out
and banishing signs of waywardness or defect, variance from prescribed norms of weight or shape, deformity or disfiguration; all of
which, under the scrutiny of the gaze, are indicative of a marked and
a lesser humanity.

This self-scrutiny, correlating closely to the 'care of the self' which
preoccupied Foucault in his later work, reflects a vital shift in social
conditions themselves, in terms of work and leisure, consumerism and
commodification, and the reflexivity implied in the project of the self
(Giddens, 1991). The body has new work to do, symbolic and social as
well as physical. At the turn of the twenty-first century, the self seems
above all a commodified self; the person is equated with their bodily
form, and in control of their appearance via the body *project* (Turner,
1984; Featherstone, 1991; Shilling 1993) with attention to this project
geared to produce preferred and fashionably desirable versions of
outward forms. This is nowhere made clearer than in media representations of the self. The late 1990s were noticeably the era of the media
'makeover': effecting changes from one kind of person-as-commodity
to another, 'better' commodity. The body in late modern societies is,
then, one of the primary loci of personal and social standing.
Maintenance and positive presentation of the body involve regimes in
pursuit of sociocultural norms of desirability that are almost invariably
focused on youth, health and beauty (Featherstone 1991, Featherstone
and Hepworth, 1990). According to Giddens's general theories, since
the self is an identity-project, and since traditional principles of social
ordering have broken down, we can 'create' ourselves, to an extent
including physically, from all manner of role-models offered to us, particularly via the media. To Giddens, then:

> The body used to be one aspect of nature, governed in a fundamen-
> tal way by processes only marginally subject to human intervention.
> The body was a 'given', the often inconvenient and inadequate seat
> of the self. With the increasing invasion of the body by abstract
> systems all this becomes altered. The body, like the self, becomes a
> site of interaction, appropriation and reappropriation, linking
> reflexively organised processes and systematically ordered expert
> knowledge ... Once thought to be the locus of the soul ... the body
> has become fully available to be 'worked upon' by the influences of

high modernity ... In the conceptual space between these, we find more and more guidebooks and practical manuals to do with health, diet, appearance, exercise, love-making and many other things. (1991: 218)

In a consumer culture, we can command the belief (ultimately illusory, but highly seductive and involving) that we can transcend the lifespan and our own ageing (Featherstone, 1991: 177). Such a belief complements Bauman's (1992) more far-reaching notion that death itself can somehow be countered through a life lived entirely in and for the present, a spurious immortality approved by the gods of consumer culture. Bodies are now themselves both subject and object, both project and projected upon, in what has been referred to as a culture of narcissism (Lasch, 1991). Like Narcissus peering into a pool and reaching out to embrace his evasive reflection, the object of attention dissolves in the space between the observer and the observed.

For Baudrillard, this narcissism, unlike the narcissism of infants, is 'planned'. One is responsible for one's own body and for investing in it, making it yield benefits, 'not in accordance with the order of enjoyment – but with the *signs* reflected and mediated by mass models, and in accordance with an organisation chart of prestige etc.' (1993: 111). The body project, as described above, is subsumed under Baudrillard's classification of tertiary or 'synthetic' narcissism, which involves a 're-writing' of the body. Under this model the body is regarded as the locus for the industrial production of signs and differences, and emphasises the 'subject's relation to its proper lack in its body, by the body which has itself become the medium of totalisation' (1993: 112). Baudrillard illustrates this overcompensating and synthetic narcissism by citing an episode in the film *Le Mépris*, in which Brigitte Bardot examines her body in a mirror, 'offering each part of it to the erotic approval of the other, the finished product being a formal addition as object: "So, d'you love every bit of me?"' (*ibid.*)

And yet narcissism exists not only as a culturally embedded affectation; it reflects an essential paradox at the heart of Cartesian dualism. If I am to be judged exclusively on the evidence of my body, how do I reconcile this with the person that my body denies me from being? This has been described, within the discipline of gerontology as 'the mask of ageing' (Featherstone and Hepworth, 1993) whereby the older person feels him/herself to be intrinsically unchanged even while the body tells (and invites) another story. In such instances the body might be compared with the Freudian unconscious, whose influence, according to psychoanalytic theory, 'the subject wishes to escape from but cannot' (Phillips, 2000: 207).

The Cartesian argument for the mind–body split contains within itself another major paradox, to do with corporeality. It was only through the body (more specifically, the pineal gland) that Descartes was able to explain the interaction of mind and body. In other words, 'it is only *because* he has defined mind quasi-corporeally or as a type of substance that he is able to effect a dualism. The problem [with Descartes] is not his negation of corporeality, but his corporealization of the mind' (Colebrook, 2000: 36). Thus the dynamics of Cartesian thought confines us to our body while at the same time suggesting that the mind (or soul) is located within that body.

Our ability to 'stand outside' our bodies even as we speak might be termed the 'othering' of the body and it is pertinent that ambiguity about what constitutes 'you' and what constitutes 'your body' is encapsulated perfectly in the nurse's question to the patient: "how are you feeling *in yourself* today?" (cf. Macleod, 1993). So the concept of a divided self, of a mind that describes (through language) the requirements and sensations of the body, and a body that is in turn projected as somehow emblematic of the mind (through its adherence to the discipline of a 'body project', for example) forms one of the substantive questions addressed in the pages that follow. If we are our bodies, and our bodies are themselves elements in the discourse of the self, then what is the relation between identity and embodiment?

With this sociocultural context as the backdrop, the twelve chapters in this book develop an account of how discourses of the body, as they are revealed in talk, text and other semiotic practices, *sustain a series of moral, ideological and practical positions*. Our intention is to show how the body is articulated as discourse, and how, in turn, discourse articulates the body. In a general sense, the theme of this book reflects its contributors' use of the term *discourse* in the broadly Foucauldian sense of one (or more) particular, internally coherent set(s) of values and orientations, which is/ are held to be normative, persuasive or simply unexceptional within specific groups or movements, which guides practical action, but which is configured around and through a finite set of claims, statements or accounts, amounting to a stance or (partial) world-view. But more specifically in terms of the analyses the contributors offer, the chapters in this book will assume not only that discourses are both ideological and textual, but that they are accessible and basically amenable to forms of linguistic, rhetorical or semiotic analysis. At least partially similar definitions or assumptions can be found in the writing of critical discourse analysts such as Candlin, Fairclough, Fowler, Hodge and Kress (Jaworski and N. Coupland, 1999).

Within this general approach, several themes emerged as the keynotes for the book.

Ideological analysis needn't be purely speculative or abstract

Until now, despite the existence of a great deal of research on the body, scholarship has tended to limit its attention to theory, with a marked lack of application of theoretical frameworks to the analysis of empirical data on the body as represented and realised in talk, text and other semiotic systems. A notable exception is Nettleton and Watson, 1998, who also cite Leder (1992) and Scott and Morgan (1993) as offering work grounded in the empirical domain. Nettleton and Watson (1998: 8–9) provide a useful review of the debate between the social constructionists (who view the body as socially created or simply an effect of discursive processes or contexts) and the anti-constructionists (or material positivists), who assume that the biological basis of the body is a universal given and impinges on our experience of the body. As they point out, most writers (see Connell, 1995; Shilling, 1993; Scott and Morgan, 1993; Turner, 1984) take up a position that argues for synthesis: framing the body as having a material biological base, but subject to alteration and modification within different social contexts. The argument for synthesis and the need for analysis of empirical data to illustrate the utility of theoretical approaches continues:

> We need to move away from the binary divide between material and discursive analyses of the body, to a position which allows us to recognise the interaction and the relationship between the two.
>
> (Ussher, 1997: 1)

The chapters in the book address this interaction and relationship by grounding their theoretical arguments in various forms of textual and semiotic analysis. This approach sees theory and data analysis as necessarily mutually informing. It is this pragmatic take which enables us to claim the book to address not 'the body as discourse' but 'discourses of the body'.

Discourse analysis must be multimodal

In line with this, the chapters in this collection examine the body at work, at play, the body experiencing change, illness, ageing, the mediated body and the body in specific social spaces and environments; and make interconnections between physical action and social interpretation. These approaches constitute an advance over traditional studies of non-verbal communication which were behaviourist and in many ways a-social/a-contextual. Here we present a diverse set of approaches, but all of them filling out the main priorities of an interactional sociolinguistics. This multimodal approach is not just evident in Part 1 on 'The Body as an Interactional Resource' (where it is, perhaps, most clearly foregrounded) but also in the chapters by Coupland, Tulloch and Tulloch, Meinhof, Jaworski, and Lupton and Seymour.

Analysis must be culturally aware

Explicit attention must be paid to cultural differences, where again there are empirical questions to be asked and answered. We take on issues of the cultural constitution of meanings of the body and bodily risk and change. This is addressed not only in respect of national communities (Meinhof) but also gender (Coupland, Tulloch and Tulloch) and disablement (Lupton and Seymour).

The body is itself not a stable phenomenon

Theoretical studies tend to abstract from socio-structural diversity. The shaping, constraining and even inventing of the body is explored by Shilling through the notion of the 'body project', with the body as 'an unfinished biological and sociological phenomenon which is changed by its participation in society; styles of walking, talking and gestures are influenced by our upbringing; the body is seen as an entity which is in the process of becoming; a project which should be worked at and accomplished as part of an individual's self-esteem' (Shilling, 1993: 5). Woodward's (1991) comments about the 'unwatchability' of old age, based on her observations of responses to fine-art portrayals of elderly nudes, is apposite. The notion of 'gerontophobia' is also relevant here, encapsulating many people's experience of reticence and even revulsion when confronted by others', and no doubt the prospect of their own, ageing. As Shilling remarks:

Investment in the body ... has its limitations. Indeed, in one sense, the effort expended by individuals on the body is doomed to failure. Bodies age and decay, and the inescapable reality of death appears particularly disturbing to modern people who are concerned with a self-identity which has at its centre the body. After all, what could signal to us more effectively the limitations of our concern with the young and fit, ideally feminine or masculine body than the brute facts of its thickening waistline, sagging flesh and inevitable death?

(1993: 7)

In this volume, the contributors address ideological values realised through different representations in the arenas of ageing and change (Hepworth, Coupland, Jaworski), the 'normal' and 'abnormal' (Lupton and Seymour, Tulloch and Tulloch and Woodward) and the nature and impact of seeking and maintaining health, and experiencing illness and disease (Gwyn, Meinhof and Woodward).

Representations and construals of the body impact directly on people's lives in the form of particular outcomes

We take it as read that the body is a routinely functioning semiotic resource. But the textual and semiotic analyses offered in this collection give access not only to the range of different representations and construals of the body, but also to the extent to which they can be shown to have tangible and practical effects on everyday lives in the form of particular outcomes (Gwyn, Lupton and Seymour).

The five themes as outlined above are addressed in variable focus by the chapters of the book, which is divided into three sections as follows:

Part 1: The body as an interactional resource

This first section explores the semiotic work of the body in its sociocultural setting; as the carrier of meaning in social interaction, through gesture, posture, proxemics and the manipulation of objects. Goodwin, and Hindmarsh and Heath show how embodied individuals are constantly taken up with the business of moving and working to construct the world around them, in constant negotiation with that world. Discourse as talk is treated here as one type of representation within a whole range of other resources which are brought to bear in order to denote, classify and index the social world.

Goodwin's chapter sees bodies first and foremost not as individuated but as engaged in multi-party interactive fields, communicating with each other and through and with the material surround. This yields an analysis of the display of meaning and action for the ongoing activity. Hindmarsh and Heath look at the animation of various objects through bodily conduct; at how the body is used to animate and illustrate features of artefacts (including bodily parts themselves); how the body is used in context to constitute the sense and significance of objects and in turn the sense and significance of the bodily interaction with that object.

Radley's chapter describes flirting in its existence as symbolic expressive activity and uses this to challenge the separation of discourse and body. Radley sees flirting as essentially not denotative but symbolically or metacommunicatively expressive and as such crucially draws on allusion and ambiguity in its practice. In this argument, the power lies in what is not stated rather than in what is. His view sees the embodied act (including talk) as a symbolic veil, wherein one particular medium of communication (verbal) must not be privileged over another (non-verbal); important ways of signifying otherwise cannot be conceptualised or described.

The work in this section shows that as analysts we need to re-embed our interpretations of talk as communication into semiotic interpretations of bodily praxis in order to see the body in all of its diversity as a social agent, incorporating talk within movement and aesthetics.

Part 2: Ideological representations of the body

The role of discourse in the social construction of the developing or changing self, the stigmatised self and the self-at-risk are the focus of the second section.

Hepworth's chapter explores the discursive realisations of the symbolic capital of the body and in particular continues his programme of work on the mask of ageing, by challenging and problematising the relationship between the ageing self and the ageing body. Against Western culture's master narrative of human ageing, which correlates diachrony and decrement, Hepworth argues that the origins of decline are not ultimately located within the body but within the social construction of ageing as inherently decremental. The force of the analysis is to shift interpretation of ageing away from the body project and towards alternative narratives, or other discursive solutions.

Tulloch and Tulloch examine the postmodern construction of bodies as sites of risk. Their focus is media representation of violent crimes which, through indicating patriarchal ideology, promulgate fear, anxiety, and outrage and thus misrepresent risk. They show how the reading of media messages is negotiated through personal experience and wider informal circuits of communication. Comparing narratives of young women on victimisation and fear of crime with those of young men, they suggest that moral tales of outrage in response to violence can play an important role in introducing revised, alternative discourses into media representations and, indeed, into public safety policies.

Coupland's chapter considers contemporary media texts as indices of sociocultural attitudes to ageing and the body project. Specifically, in print media advertisements and features on skin care, facial and bodily appearance of ageing is framed as degeneration, and as correctable aberration. This reveals a gendered and consumerised aspect of bodily commodification deriving from contemporary Western culture's belief in youth and beauty as dominating women's symbolic capital. Coupland examines how skincare products are marketed and given authenticity using discourses derived from medicine and pharmacy. In addition, these consumerised discourses encourage the bodily project of 'safe tanning', a contested discourse which attempts to offset ageing and environmental risk discourses against discourses of consumerism, desire, style and bodily display.

The next two chapters examine the 'normal' body and its actions and activities as contested practice and raise questions about what constitutes normality and deviance. Jaworski's chapter gives us access to the self-commentaries of lay individuals speaking of their own bodies, which enables examination of the range of discourses drawn on to extemporise on corporeality. These representations of the embodied self reveal both conformity and little rebellions, and display individuals' discursive struggles about fitting the perceived reality of the body with socioculturally expressed ideals in relation to ageing, gender and sexuality, and aesthetics. Dominant ideologies of the body are at times aligned with, but there are also discourses which subvert and challenge those dominant ideologies.

Meinhof's chapter addresses the body in its cultural setting, and examines ways of making displays and settings for this cultural body. A cross-cultural ethnographic analysis examines, first, the discourses involved in and representing sauna provision and facilities (semiotic systems, incorporating spatial, decorative and other visual messages) and, secondly, ways in which the norms and expectations of usage are communicated via notices, pictures and promotional leaflets. The construction of the body which emerges from these discourses reflects how naked or partially clothed bodies in the sauna are positioned within the social world; as variably healthy, leisurely, sexual and illicit across different social and cultural contexts.

Part 3: The body, pathology and constructions of selfhood

This last section takes us into the realms of the damaged, threatened and stigmatised body: subject to science and medicine as dominant ideologies. Here, bodily problems set the body as the property of the individual against the body as an institutional phenomenon, rendered part of social arrangements. In this section we see individuals attempting to use their discursive resources to make sense of, or to come to terms with, the bodily experience of themselves or of others.

Gwyn's chapter traces individuals using discourse as a resource for sense-making in their living through life-threatening illness. His analysis of biographical accounts of cancer experiences examines how the individual may literally write a refiguration of her/his identity via the embodied changes the illness forces them to experience. Body, self and society are challenged and re-examined from a new perspective, a new identity of the cancer patient. The self, to the author, often becomes a stigmatised 'other', forcing a body–self separation. The 'sense-making struggles' that he observes lead him to argue that illness narrative is an ideal focus for study of the expression of embodied thought.

Woodward's chapter again uses illness narratives, but here to examine the statistical body as the body of risk, using mediated data, from a popular television drama, an independent film and a memoir. Woodward examines how contemporary cultural texts contribute to, dissect, confront and reject the statistical body. She asks how the depersonalising statistics of bodily risk can achieve real meaning for and understanding by individuals by setting statistical discourses, or scientific use of the language of risk, against the stories of the victims of illness, living risk in the experiential dimension.

Lupton and Seymour challenge the ubiquity of normality as established by the 'healthy' fully able body. Their chapter explores the interaction between embodiment, subjectivity and disability. Reflexive commentaries by disabled individuals allow the authors to explore how the 'othering' experienced by people with disabilities obscures or eliminates consideration of other aspects of the self or the body. They also give us access to understanding how individuals with disabilities can maintain a highly meaningful yet disembodied or alternatively embodied self via use of new communication technologies.

In what ways, then, might the essays contained within this volume be considered to advance the study of embodiment, identity and the self? First, each of the chapters here adopts what might broadly be described as a discourse analytic approach, based on an eclectic brew of data examples of interaction and bodily display, self-reports in interviews, advertising materials and signs, media news reporting, film and TV shows, narratives and biographies. The authors are able to engage more thoroughly with the notion of embodiment than might be the case in a more theoretically driven study. This is not to minimise the importance of theory in debates surrounding embodiment and identity, but to argue that theory is better served by being complemented with examples from the world of lived experience, with a view to asserting those moral, ideological and practical positions we enumerated above.

Secondly, the diversity of themes and topics, while falling under the three broad categories into which we have divided the book, indicates not only the enormous potential of the study of embodiment in relation to identity and selfhood, but also, paradoxically, some kind of commonality of intent, given the wide-ranging approaches the contributors have taken to the body 'topics' under scrutiny. Our contributing authors make different methodological assumptions which lead them to take different analytic approaches, ranging from (in no particular order) ethnomethodology/conversation analysis through semiotic analysis, post-structural analysis, ethnography of communication to critical discourse analysis. Ideas and theoretical frameworks from sociolinguistics, pragmatics, sociology, psychology, anthropology, critical and cultural theory all add to the mix. But it would be oversimplistic to characterise individual chapters as, in all cases, representing distinctive (or easily distinguishable) perspectives, as the chapters' reference lists show. It is, after all, as Rajagopalan (1999: 449) reminds us, one of the aims of discourse analysis to be ready to 'cross indeed *transgress* disciplinary boundaries if need be, so as to explore solutions to given problems, regardless of from which discipline the best solutions may be forthcoming'.

In addition, as Schegloff has pointed out (1997: 171), where several approaches are invited to come together 'each tends to choose texts that best illustrate its proponents' views'. It is no accident then, in our own cases for example, that Coupland's methodological preference for critical discourse analysis with its emphasis on the ideological force of texts leads her to work on media discourses on the body that arguably constitute and perpetuate gender and age prejudices, or that Gwyn's preference for narrative analysis should seek out accounts of chronic illness experience that often convey a mythopoeic vision of the self. Thus, a range of approaches to discourse, the body and identity come together in one volume. Wetherell's (1998) contribution to the debate about discourse and the 'appropriate' methodological framework for its analysis (a debate most notably ignited by Schegloff, 1997) seems apposite here. Wetherell (1998: 392–3) cites Laclau and Mouffe (1987) who 'conceive the social space as a whole as discursive. Or, as Laclau (1993: 341) puts it: '*[s]ociety can ... be understood as a vast argumentative texture through which people construct their reality*'. Laclau is at pains to stress that the argumentative fabric from which social realities are constructed is both verbal and non-verbal: '*there is ... an unceasing human activity of making meanings (the horizon of discourse) from which social agents and objects, social institutions and social structures emerge configured in ever-changing patterns of relations*'. And, as Wetherell comments later, '[a]nalysis works by *carving out a piece of the argumentative social fabric for closer examination*' (our italics). As we have commented above, little published work on the body up to this point is data-led in its attention to the discourse–body–identity relationship. So Wetherell's argument above seems nicely to capture the enormity and range of the enterprise that discourse analysts are engaged in. To extend Wetherell's metaphor, we see the contributors here as carving their chosen pieces of social fabric and using a variety of conceptual lenses (Tracy and Naughton, 2000) to examine their texture, their warp and woof.

Readers will, of course, come to this volume with their own favoured theoretical frameworks, their own methodological preferences, and their own reasons for engaging with and in discourse. To each, some of the approaches used here will have a comfortable 'fit' with their own intellectual preferences; some will challenge, some may open up new ideas and possibilities. The contributions to this collection serve to illustrate the realignment of traditional disciplines within the social sciences, and this in itself, in our view, constitutes advancement. And the conclusions drawn in this book, while by no means progressing uniformly towards a cohesive theory of embodiment, work towards, if not *a* theory, then multiple interconnecting and complementary perspectives on the way that we envision, represent and invest in our bodies in the course of everyday living.

Note

We would like to thank an anonymous reviewer for her/his comments on an earlier version of this chapter.

Selected references

Baudrillard, J. (1993) *Symbolic Exchange and Death*. London: Sage.
Bauman, Z. (1992) *Mortality, Immortality, and Other Life Strategies*. Stanford: Stanford University Press.
Candlin, C. (1997) General editor's preface. In B.-L.Gunnarsson, P. Linnell and B. Nordberg (eds) *The Construction of Professional Discourse*. London: Longman, pp. ix–xiv.
Cole, T.R. and Gadow, S. (eds) (1986) *What Does It Mean to Grow Old? Reflections from the Humanities*. Durham, NC: Duke University Press.
Colebrook, C. (2000) 'Incorporeality: The Ghostly Body of Metaphysics'. *Body and Society* 6(2): 25–44.
Connell, R.W. (1995) *Masculinities*. Cambridge: Polity Press.
Fairclough, N. (1992) 'Discourse and Text: Linguistic and Intertextual Analysis within Discourse Analysis'. *Discourse and Society* 3(2): 193–217.
Featherstone, M. (1991) 'The Body in Consumer Culture'. In M. Featherstone, M. Hepworth and B. Turner (eds) *The Body: Social Process and Cultural Theory*. London: Sage, 170–96.
Featherstone, M. and Hepworth, M. (1990) 'Images of Ageing'. In J. Bond and P. Coleman (eds) *Ageing in Society: An Introduction to Social Gerontology*. London: Sage, 250–75.
Foucault, M. (1973) *The Birth of the Clinic*. London: Tavistock.
Foucault, M. (1977) *Discipline and Punish: the Birth of the Prison*. Harmondsworth: Penguin.
Foucault, M. (1979) *The History of Sexuality*, vol. 1. Harmondsworth: Penguin.
Fowler, R. (1981) *Literature as Social Discourse: The Practice of Linguistic Criticism*. London: Batsford Academic.
Giddens, A. (1991) *Modernity and Self-identity; Self and Society in the Late Modern Age*. Cambridge: Polity Press.
Goffman, E. (1959) *The Presentation of Self in Everyday Life*. Harmondsworth: Penguin.
Goffman, E. (1968) *Stigma: Notes on the Management of Spoiled Identity*. Harmondsworth: Penguin.
Greer, G. (1991) *The Change: Women, Ageing and the Menopause*. London: Hamish Hamilton.
Gwyn, R. (2002) *Communicating Health and Illness*. London: Sage.
Hall, S. (1996) 'Introduction: Who Needs "Identity"?' In S. Hall and P. du Gay (eds) *Questions of Cultural Identity*. London: Sage.
Hodge, R. and Kress, G. (1991) *Social Semiotics*. Cambridge: Polity.
Illich, I. (1976) *Limits to Medicine: Medical Nemesis: The Expropriation of Health*. London: Marion Boyars.
Jamieson, A., Harper, S. and Victor, C. (eds) (1997) *Critical Approaches to Ageing and Later Life*. Buckingham: Open University Press.
Jaworski, A. and Coupland, N. (eds) (1999) *The Discourse Reader*. London: Routledge.

Laclau, E. and Mouffe, C. (1987) 'Post-Marxism without Apologies', *New Left Review* 166: 79–106.

Laclau, E. (1993) 'Politics and the Limits of Modernity', in T. Docherty (ed.) *Postmodernism: A Reader*. London: Harvester Wheatsheaf, 329–44.

Lasch, C. (1991) *The Culture of Narcissism*. New York: Norton.

Leder, D. (1992) Introduction. In D. Leder (ed.) *The Body in Medical Thought and Practice*. London: Kluwer Academic.

Lupton, D. (1994) *Medicine as Culture*. London: Sage.

Macleod, M. (1993) 'On Knowing the Patient: Experiences of Nurses Undertaking Care'. In A. Radley (ed.) *Worlds of Illness*. London: Routledge.

May, W.F. (1986) 'The Virtues and Vices of the Elderly'. In Cole and Gadow (eds) *What Does It Mean to Grow Old?*, 41–62.

Nettleton, S. and Watson, J. (eds) (1998) *The Body in Everyday Life*. London: Routledge.

Phillips, A. (2000) *Promises, Promises: Essays on Literature and Psychoanalysis*. London: Faber & Faber.

Rajagopalan, K. (1999) 'Discourse Analysis and the Need for Being Critical All the Way Through' *Discourse and Society* 10(3): 449–51.

Scott, S. and Morgan, D. (eds) (1993) *Body Matters: Essays on the Sociology of the Body*. London: The Falmer Press.

Schegloff, E. (1997) 'Whose Text? Whose Context?' *Discourse and Society* 8(2): 165–87.

Shilling, C. (1993) *The Body and Social Theory*. London: Sage.

Tracy, K. and Naughton, J.M. (2000) 'Institutional Identity Work: A Better Lens'. In J. Coupland (ed.) *Small Talk*. London: Pearson Education.

Turner, B.S. (1984) *The Body and Society*. Oxford: Blackwell.

Turner, B.S. (1995) 'Ageing and Identity: Some Reflections on the Somatization of the Self'. In Featherstone and Wernick (eds) *Images of Ageing*, 245–62.

Ussher, J.M. (ed.) (1997) *Body Talk: The Material and Discursive Regulation of Sexuality, Madness and Reproduction*, London: Routledge.

Wetherell, M. (1998) 'Positioning and Interpretative Repertoires: Conversation Analysis and Post-structuralism in Dialogue'. *Discourse and Society* 9(3): 387–412.

Woodward, K. (1991) *Aging and Its Discontents: Freud and Other Fictions*. Bloomington, IN: Indiana University Press.

Part 1

The Body as an Interactional Resource

2
The Body in Action

Charles Goodwin

This chapter will use videotapes of young archaeologists learning how to see and excavate the traces of an ancient village in the soil they are digging to explore some of the ways in which the human body is implicated in the structuring of human language, cognition and social organisation. Clearly the part played by the body in such processes can be analysed from a number of different perspectives. One can focus, for example, on how experiencing the world through a brain embedded in a body structures human cognition (Damasio, 1994; 1999). Such a perspective provides a counter to theories that treat cognition as the disembodied manipulation of symbolic structures, and places the body in the world at the centre of much contemporary thinking about the neural infrastructure of cognitive processes (Rizzolatti and Arbib, 1998). Moreover, it sheds light on pervasive processes that shape how the symbols that human beings construct emerge from forms of experience that have a crucial embodied component (Johnson, 1987; Lakoff and Johnson, 1999). For example, the universal experience of bodies situated within a gravitational field leads in all languages and cultures to a range of metaphors that contrast high and low or up and down (for example the symbols used to describe social hierarchies). However, it is possible to focus such analysis of embodiment largely or entirely on the experience of what is in fact an isolated individual, for example to investigate how being in a body shapes cognition and consciousness. What results is a rich analysis of psychological processes, but one in which other bodies, and social processes play only a minor, peripheral role. By way of contrast, in this chapter I want to investigate how multiple participants take each other's bodies into account as they build relevant action in concert with each other. Moreover, human bodies, and the actions they are visibly performing, are situated within a consequential setting. The positioning, actions, and orientation of the body in the environment are crucial to how participants understand what is happening and build action together. In this chapter, embodiment will be investigated as a central component of the public practices used to build action within situated human interaction.

Symbiotic gestures

We'll begin by examining a particular type of gesture. The following provides an example. It occurred during one of the first days of an archaeological field school. Ann, the senior archaeologist and director of the school, is helping a young graduate student use the point of her trowel to outline a pattern visible in the soil they are excavating, in this case the hole that contained one of the posts that held up an ancient building. Sue is having difficulty in determining where exactly to draw the line. In line 19 Ann suggests that she remove some of the soil at a particular place ('in the:re' accompanied by a gesture over the place being indicated). When Sue hesitates, Ann repeats the request in line 21 by saying 'Toward you around parallel'. As she says 'around parallel' Ann puts her index finger just above the area in the soil being talked about and moves it in an arc over the area being specified (in essence tracing the pattern in the soil that Sue is being asked to trowel in the air above it). The gesture is repeated in the silence just after her utterance, as indicated in Figure 2.1.

Most analysis of gesture focuses on the movements of the speaker's body, typically the hand. However, neither Sue, nor anyone else, could see the action that Ann is performing here just by attending to her hand. What Sue must see if she is to understand Ann's action in a relevant fashion is not a only a gesture, but the patterning in the earth she is being instructed to follow. The soil under Ann's finger is indispensable to the action complex being built here. The finger indicates relevant graphic structure in the soil (that is, the patterning of the post mould they are trying to outline), while simultaneously that structure provides organisation for the precise location, shape and trajectory of the gesture. Each mutually elaborates the other (and both are further elaborated by the talk that accompanies the gesture). I'll call action complexes of this type *Symbiotic Gestures*. The term Symbiotic is meant to capture the way in which a whole that is both different from, and greater than its parts, is constructed through the mutual interdependence of unlike elements.

19 Ann: En maybe trowel just a little bit in the:re.
20   (1.5)

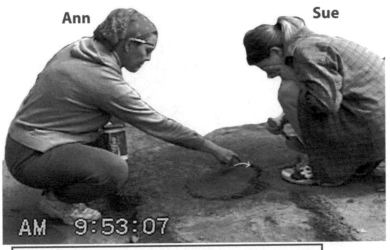

21 Ann: Toward you around para:llel.

Figure 2.1

Analogy with a game, such as football, might make more clear what is meant by this. If one were to look just at the body of a runner moving a ball (Figure 2.2), one would see his or her movements and the path they made.

However, these movements could not be understood by looking at the runner's body in isolation. Instead, they are given organisation through their positioning on the visible graphic structure of the playing-field (Figure 2.3).

Thus, moving over the line at the end of the field constitutes a touchdown or goal, an action that does not occur when the runner moves over the other lines on the field. To perform relevant action in the game, a body must use structures that are located outside itself. The runner's body is given meaning by the contextual field it is embedded within. Similarly, while the playing-field contains the semiotic and physical resources that will make possible particular kinds of action (goals, firstdowns, and so on), these actions can only come into being when bodies move through the field as part of a game. Each requires the other. The runner's movements are also organised with an eye

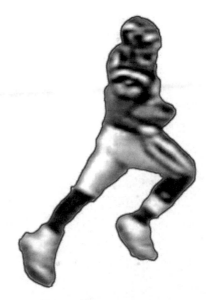

Figure 2.2

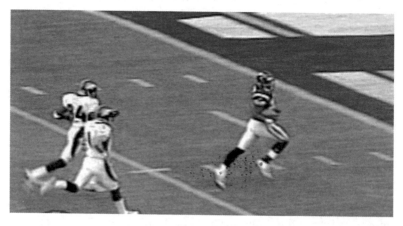

Figure 2.3

toward the movements and actions of others on the field. With these structures in place, relevant aspects of the mental life of the runner, for instance his intention to move toward a particular place on the field, such as the goal-line, are immediately visible to all present, and indeed have a public organisation. In short, rather than being lodged in a single modality, such as the body, talk, or structure in the environment, many forms of human action are built through the juxtaposition of quite diverse materials, including the actor's body, the bodies of others, language, structure in the environment, and so on. Moreover, because of the medium they are embedded within, each of these resources has very different properties. The gestalt pattern of a graphic field, and the ability to see the relevance of continuously changing movement within it, is quite unlike the emergence of an utterance as a successive sequence of discrete events through time. Elsewhere (Goodwin, 2000a) I have investigated in more detail how action can be not only built, but continuously changed and updated by assembling diverse semiotic fields into contextual configurations that are relevant to the activities that participants are pursuing in a particular setting.

In an analogous fashion, symbiotic gestures are built through the conjunction of quite different kinds of entity instantiated in diverse media: first, talk; second, gesture; and third, material and graphic structure in the environment. The actions they are performing cannot be understood by focusing on the gesturing hand in isolation, or even just on the gesture and the talk that accompanies it. Symbiotic gestures might thus constitute one perspicuous site for investigating embodiment as something lodged within both human interaction and a consequential, structured environment.

In many environments symbiotic gestures are very frequent, indeed pervasive. In a 2-minute 49-second strip of interaction that included the talk being analysed here, I counted 34 symbiotic gestures. Such figures provide at least a rough demonstration that gesturing activity of this type can be frequent, indeed pervasive, in some types of interaction. For other common examples of such gestural practices consider computer screens smeared with finger prints, television weather forecasts, or pointing at overheads during academic talks.

Symbiotic gestures would thus seem to constitute a common, indeed major, class of gestural activity. In light of this it is striking that symbiotic gestures have received little sustained analysis by students of gesture (but see Hutchins and Palen, 1997; Nevile, 2001). A major reason for this would seem to lie in the nature of the theoretical frameworks that have been developed for the analysis of gesture. One, well exemplified in the work of David McNeill and his colleagues (McNeill, 1992), analyses gesture as an embodied manifestation of the same psychological processes that lead to the production of sentences and utterances. This work provides important analysis of a host of phenomena implicated in the mutual relationship of language and gesture.

However, in that its analytic point of departure is processes inside the mind of the individual speaker/gesturer, this approach does not provide the resources necessary for investigating how phenomena outside the speaker, for example a consequential physical environment, contribute to the organisation of gesture.

A second important approach to gesture focuses on how it is organised within human interaction (Goodwin, 1986; Heath, 1986; Kendon, 1980, 1986, 1990a, 1997; LeBaron and Streeck, 2000; Schegloff, 1984; Streeck, 1993, 1994). This research has provided detailed analytic resources for demonstrating how gesture is consequential to the organisation of action in human interaction, and how participants other than the gesturer (for example addressees and other kinds of hearers) are central to its organisation. However, in much of this work, including my own, little attention is paid to how structure in the environment contributes to the organisation of gesture. In essence an analytic boundary is drawn at the skin of the participants. The neglect of symbiotic gesture, despite its pervasiveness, might thus arise from the fact that while existing approaches to the study of gesture provide units of analysis that include the psychology, distinctive culture (Kendon, 1995), bodies, and interaction of the participants, they do not encompass phenomena in the environment, such as the soil in example 1.[1] In short, symbiotic gestures seem to slip beyond the traditional classifications of gesture in that they include not only movements of a speaker's body, but also something outside the body: structure in the surround. This neglect is, however, being rectified. Analysis of phenomena such as symbiotic gestures contributes to an important stream of current research on gesture which investigates how gesture is tied to the physical, semiotic, social and cultural properties of the environment within which it is embedded (Haviland, 1995, 1998; Haviland, 1996; Heath and Hindmarsh, 2000; Heath and Luff, 1996; Hindmarsh and Heath in press; Hindmarsh and Heath, this volume; LeBaron, 1998; LeBaron and Streeck, 2000; Nevile, 2001).

Do the participants themselves attend to the distinctive structure of symbiotic gestures and treat it as consequential to the activities they are engaged in? The talk that occurs in line 21 'Toward you around para:llel' is grammatically incomplete. Parallel lacks a complement. Sue is not told just what her trowelling should be parallel to. Both speakers and hearers have well-developed practices for displaying to each other that there are problems in a particular utterance (Goodwin, 1981, 1987; Goodwin and Goodwin, 1986; Jefferson, 1974; Schegloff, 1979, 1992; Schegloff *et al.*, 1977). None of these practices are used here;

instead the utterance is spoken with untroubled fluency and Ann's addressee does not treat what's said here as incomplete or lacking something. Such unproblematic treatment of this talk, despite its grammatical anomaly, is not, of course, mysterious. Both participants can clearly see what the trowelling should be parallel to: the patterning in the soil located by the symbiotic gesture.

One thus finds here an utterance in which not only talk but also structure in the environment and gesture linking the two are central to its organisation. If these were removed, what was being said would not be expressed, and the action being performed would fail. The symbiotic gesture is thus most consequential in that the speaker displays in the construction of her utterance that she expects her addressee not only to see it, but take it into account as a crucial component of the process of locating just what is being said, and the action it is requesting.

Defining a feature

The actions being investigated here link the body to both language and an environment that is the visible focus of participants' current orientation and activity. Why might action packages with such a structure be so useful to participants that they occur pervasively in certain settings? To investigate this issue it is necessary to look more closely at the activities that Ann and Sue are pursuing. Sue, a new archaeologist, is faced with the task of mastering the practices required to reliably transform the raw materials provided by the soil being excavated into the signs and categories that constitute archaeology as a discipline (for example maps of structures, such as the outline of a house, the location and categorisation of relevant cultural artefacts, and so on). In so far as the ability to see such structure in the soil is not an idiosyncratic, individual accomplishment, but instead part of the professional vision expected of any competent archaeologist, such seeing must be organised as a form of public practice. Actions, such as symbiotic gestures, that link the actual soil in all of its complexity to relevant archaeological categories within systematic work practices, provide excellent resources for negotiating shared vision within a consequential public arena. Moreover, rather than simply providing definitions of categories, the process of using such talk and gesture to actually work with the soil being excavated helps organise the ensemble of embodied practices required to competently locate in 'nature' the soil being investigated, valid instances of such categories, and transform them into the signs (maps, names, and so on) required for further work with them.

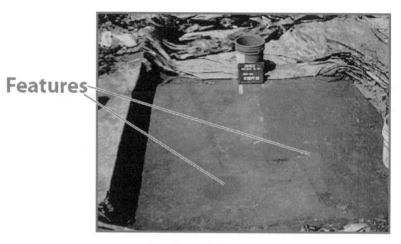

Figure 2.4

We will now look more closely at what Ann and Sue are doing, and the larger activities within which their work is embedded. The sequences being examined were recorded during one of the very first days of an archaeological field school. The participants are engaged in an activity that they call *Defining a Feature*. Many phenomena of interest to archaeologists, what they call *features*, are visible only as colour-changes in the soil they are excavating. For example, the cinders produced by an ancient hearth will leave a black stain and the decaying material in an old post hole will produce a tube of soil, called a post mould, with colour significantly different from the soil around it (Figure 2.4).

The very activity of excavating features systematically destroys them. As soil is removed to dig deeper, the patterns of visible colour difference are destroyed. In part because of this, careful records, including maps, photographs and coding forms of various types have to be made at each stage of the excavation. A map of a set of features can reveal the pattern of an ancient structure (see Figure 2.5).

In the data being investigated here, a young archaeologist is learning how to outline the colour differences that mark the presence of a post mould in the soil. This is being done to prepare that shape so that it can be transferred to a map (indeed an earlier version of the simplified map in Figure 2.5). In the abstract this process might appear both simple (just trace a pattern visible in the soil being excavated) and of little theoretical interest. However, it is here that the soil being exca-

Determining what counts as cultural (and thus something to be recorded and brought back to the lab in some fashion) is by no means an automatic, or even easy task. For example, the site being excavated in the data being examined here had been successively occupied by a number of different social groups. The land is in the American South. The excavation is focusing on the remains of a large Native American city. The archaeologists strongly suspect that it is in fact a particular city that was described by the first European expedition into the area as being ruled by a powerful woman leader. After conquest by the Europeans, the land became part of a very large plantation with many slaves. One of the most famous diaries of the civil war was written there by a wife of its owner who described herself as living in an African village (and, indeed, since new slaves were arriving in this state even during the civil war it is likely that the slaves in fact included people who had been born in Africa). The land was subsequently bought by a rich industrial family who continue to farm it today. Ploughing the soil will, of course, disturb archaeological features if the plough reaches deep enough into the soil. Many other natural processes, such as burrowing animals, will also disturb the soil. When the owner of the farm learned that it contained an important archaeological site, he tried to protect the site by no longer ploughing it to plant crops, but instead covering it with pine trees. This had disastrous effects since the roots of the trees burrow deeply into the soil. A work crew of Mexican migrant workers planted the trees in a single day. Though Latin American workers were used extensively in this state as farm labourers, they largely lived in migrant camps (in sometimes appalling conditions) far from towns and cities and most people were unaware of their presence. The site itself had been partially excavated on several occasions by earlier teams of archaeologists, and indeed the current excavation is the latest stage in a long-term project.

The soil being excavated thus contains traces of the labour and activities of many different social groups: Native Americans, slaves working on a plantation in the American South, later farmers, Latin American workers, earlier archaeologists, and so on. In order to see and accurately map the features that are the focus of her work, a young archaeologist must navigate a complex perceptual environment. For example, the features she is trying to outline may be hidden or deformed by later ploughing, an activity that leaves its own quite visible patterning in the soil (note the long stripe beginning at the top left of the excavation in Figure 2.4). Such plough scars are, of course, the visible traces of farming, an important earlier cultural activity. However, though they are carefully mapped, such plough scars are not considered cultural materials to be analysed as part of the Native American site but instead are treated as *disturbances* which obscure and deform the features that the archaeologist wants to uncover (and thus for the purposes at hand equivalent to natural disturbance that would result from the activities of burrowing animals). Thus, in order to see features, the archaeologist must not only learn to recognise a range of other kinds of object as well, but must also take into account how they might have changed what she is trying to reveal, and make relevant judgements as to just what subset of visible cultural activities are to count as features of the structures being excavated.

The work of locating a feature involves not only culturally organised vision, but an ensemble of other embodied practices as well. To remove soil, the archaeologist scrapes away soil with the side of her trowel. As she does this she is sensitive to the feel of the soil, and to sounds, and so on, that might indicate that a solid object, or different kind of soil is being encountered. When a feature, say a roughly circular post mould, is encountered, the work with the trowel is changed: instead of scraping in a constant direction, say right across the feature, the archaeologist attempts to trowel around its contours so as to remove soil from it without damaging it. Where and how the trowel is used is thus shaped by a developing expectation about what it is uncovering, while the way in which the trowel structures the visibility of the soil helps to further clarify that very object.

Archaeologists call the process of revealing in the soil the colour patterning that marks a relevant cultural entity, and then drawing a line with a trowel that outlines its shape, 'Defining a Feature'. This expression captures very well the way in which a feature as a semiotic object (such as something that is categorised by a particular social group as a particular kind of entity and marked on a map) emerges as the product of both actual patterning in the soil being investigated, and the cultural categories and embodied practices used by archaeologists to make it visible as a particular kind of phenomenal object.

Drawing attention to the way in which the objects in the world that are studied by scientists are shaped, and constructed in part through cultural practices, is sometimes argued to demonstrate that these objects do not 'really' exist. Nothing could be further from the truth for the archaeological objects being investigated here, which are continually probed through explicit socially organised practice. Moreover, the archaeologists themselves, more than any outside observer, are acutely aware that their categories might be in error. For example, posts are constructed from trees, and indeed a tree can leave traces in the soil that closely resemble a post mould. Students are told that they could well get to the bottom of what they have been digging as a post mould and find roots extending from it, and thus discover that they have not in fact been excavating a cultural feature. The categorisations they have made can not only be challenged by others, but overturned by the world they are probing.

The bodies around a gesture

The forms of embodiment relevant to the action being constructed here extend far beyond the speaker's gesturing hand. Thus, gestures are contextualised by participation frameworks constituted through the embodied mutual orientation of the participants within an interaction. For example, in Figure 2.6, Ann gazes toward her gesturing hand and the soil it is tied to. The gesture is visibly and publicly what she is attending to, and thus something that others should take into account if they want to co-participate in action with her, or understand what she is saying and doing.

At the same time Ann's gesture is also organised with reference to the visible orientation of her addressee's body. The gesturing hand is

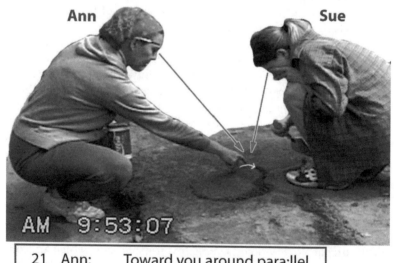

| 21 | Ann: | Toward you around para:llel. |

Figure 2.6

placed right in Sue's line of sight. It is designed not only to express what the speaker is saying, but quite literally to show Sue something, and moreover to insist that Sue look at it by intruding into her visual focus on the soil she is working with.

Such contextualisation of gesture by the bodies of multiple parties implicated in the action it is performing has a number of consequences. First, it is quite clear that not all gestures are organised to be explicitly communicative (for example, designed, as this one is, so that an addressee will take it into account). This is in no way surprising. The hand is one of the main ways that the human body explores and knows the world in all of its complexity. It is to be expected that movements of the hand will be part and parcel of the way in which speakers think and talk about the world. However, the fact that hearers frequently show no evidence of attending a speaker's gestures is sometimes argued to show that gestures are not in fact communicative (Krauss *et al.*, 1991; Rimé and Schiaratura, 1991). However, when the contextualising displays of other parts of the body are taken into account it becomes clear that not all gestures are the same. By gazing toward a gesturing hand, and/or using deictics that explicitly direct attention to the gesture (Goodwin, 1986; Streeck, 1994), a speaker can instruct the hearer to take it into account. The placement of gestures in an addressee's line of sight constitutes a complementary aspect of this process. Such practices help locate, not only for analysts, but also for participants, a class of gestures that are clearly built to be communicative.

Second, within a single action there can in fact be a number of quite different kinds of embodiment that are relevant to its organisation. Ann's gaze towards her hand and the soil underneath it is not a gesture, but something quite different, a way of publicly displaying the current focus of her orientation and action. Moreover, her gaze is embedded within a larger postural configuration that is also displaying her current orientation to Sue's work in the soil in front of them. This postural configuration has dynamic organisation of its own. Kendon (1990b) has noted that within interaction the different segments of the body provide participants with resources for making a hierarchal cluster of displays about their involvement in the events of the moment. The lower body can remain comparatively fixed for extended strips of interaction, and thus display continuing orientation towards other co-participants or relevant phenomena in the surround. Within this larger display the upper body can move in different directions and mark changing shifts in alignment. The bodily displays of separate participants are organised into multi-party participation frameworks

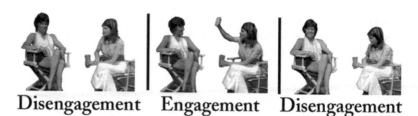

Figure 2.7

(Goodwin, 1981; Goodwin, 1997). Thus a continuing state of talk can be marked by spates of focused engagement interspaced with periods of temporary disengagement (Goodwin, 1981: 95–125; 2002). Throughout this process the lower body marks a pattern of orientation that sustains the encounter, while the upper body marks shifting alignment within it (see Figure 2.7).

Gesturing hands, changing facial displays and talk constitute not only the most dynamic level of this set of nested sign systems being displayed by the body, but also the place where participants explicitly focus their attention.

Though all of these displays may be performed simultaneously by a single body (or set of bodies when viewed from the perspective of participation frameworks), it is crucial to remember that what is occurring is not a single form of embodiment, but instead sets of signs that differ from each other significantly in their structure, organisation and relevance. For example, gestures differ markedly from the orientation display made by the lower body. Thus each kind of display has a quite different scope and duration. Gestures typically occur within the space of a single utterance, while a postural configuration being sustained by the lower body can endure over extended strips of interaction. Moreover, the referential content of these signs is quite different. Gestures typically refer to what is being talked about, while participation displays are about the interaction itself. They create a spatial and temporal boundary, an 'ecological huddle' (Goffman, 1964), within which an arena for mutual orientation, shared attention to a common environment and collaborative action can be constituted. Despite such differences these diverse forms of embodiment are used in conjunction with each other to build relevant action. Thus gestures are organised as communicative actions through the way in which they are embedded within the patterns of mutual orientation made visible through embodied participation displays.

The symbiotic gesture that Ann uses to tell Sue what to do in line 21 is thus made salient and relevant through the way in which it is embedded within a constellation of other kinds of display being made by the participants' bodies.

Symbiotic gestures and inscription

A second action occurred during this sequence that is intimately related to symbiotic gestures (see Goodwin, in press). During line 58 in Figure 2.8, Sue performs a symbiotic gesture, moving her trowel just above the soil, tracing where she sees the boundaries of a feature. When Ann agrees, Sue's hand performs this movement again (line 62). However, she now lowers the point of her trowel into the soil so that an enduring line marking the outline is left there (images on the right).

By lowering her trowel into the soil as she moves her hand Sue transduces the shape that is the focus of her gesture from one medium (the moving hand) into another (the soil itself). Through this process the gesture leaves a permanent trace on the environmental field it is highlighting and describing. This will be called *Inscription.*[2]

It might be argued that these two hand movements are quite different kinds of action: the first, a gesture, and the second, something else, a form of drawing that, unlike the gesture, actually changes the world being talked about. However, Sue's second movement is not something

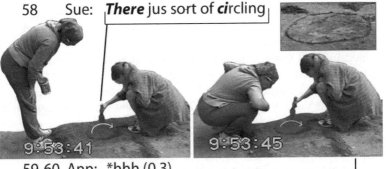

58   Sue: ***There*** jus sort of ci**r**cling

9:53:41   9:53:45

59-60   Ann: *hhh (0.3)
61   Yeah. do you see: r:righ⌈t ta he:re.
62   Sue: ⌊Right the:re.
63-64   Ann: ***Yeah Goo:d.*** (0.2) Goo:d.

Figure 2.8

entirely different, but a slight modification of the first. It thus seems more appropriate and useful analytically to follow the participants and treat these two events as points on a continuum that includes, for example, iconic gestures that in no way invoke the immediate surround, symbiotic gestures, and here gestures that act upon and transform what they are representing. Rather than constituting a tightly bounded domain of phenomena, gesture is implicated in varied ways in a range of practices through which bodies know, think about and act upon the world.

Embodied framing of an intersubjective field

As in the data examined earlier, Sue's gestures do not stand alone, but instead are embedded within a matrix of other signs being displayed by not only her body, but also her addressee's. She performs both gestures right where Ann is looking within a participation framework that establishes joint focus on the soil being worked with. More crucially, the symbiotic gestures constitute the focal actions in the exchanges that occur here. Thus, in line 58 (Figure 2.8) Sue is using the gesture to show Ann where she thinks the feature is located. Ann's agreement is what sets off the act of inscription, or in terms of the archaeological activity in progress, the drawing of the line that defines that feature. Ann's encouraging comments in lines 63–64 are not responsive to anything that is being said, but instead to the accuracy with which Sue's inscription is following the outline of the feature. Her talk here presupposes a particular kind of speaker, one who is intently following the actions of her co-participant's hand as it works within the structured field of a relevant environment, here the soil. Rather than constituting something that can be ignored, the gestures that occur here are central to the actions that these participants are engaged in, and are done precisely so that the other can take them into account.

This same point is demonstrated in a different way in Figure 2.9. In line 7 Ann uses a symbiotic gesture, tracing a circular path over a particular place in the soil, to show Sue where to draw. In response Sue brings her trowel to exactly where Ann had been pointing (in fact there is almost a collision between Sue's trowel and Ann's finger) and starts to draw:

By drawing where she does Sue not only demonstrates that she has seen Ann's gesture, and taken it into account, but that the gesture is in fact the point of departure for her response to Ann (which is done through the action of drawing the outline of the feature rather than

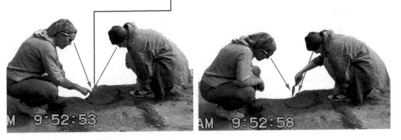

7 Ann: **Light**ly ⌐draw this in since you can see it. ⌐

8-9 Sue: Okay. (1.8)
10-13 Ann: Yeah. (0.6) Yeah. I like it.

Figure 2.9

talk). Their hands exchange places over the same spot in the soil. Then, as Sue draws, Ann produces talk that is responsive to what she sees Ann doing.

An ecology of sign systems

From a slightly different perspective, what occurs here sheds light on the relationship between language and gesture as different kinds of sign system that can function together to build relevant action. Rather than telling Ann where to draw, Ann shows her with a symbiotic gesture linked to talk describing what should be done there. Consider how difficult it would be to describe the precise place where this shape was located through language alone, and how easy it is with gesture linked to the area being talked about. As a system capable of building a potentially limitless set of discrete signs by combining and recombining a smaller set of conventional elements language has enormous power. In Bateson's (1972) terms language is digitial, while gestures (at least those being examined here) are analogic (for example they achieve their effects through continuous variation, iconicity and proximity). Despite its combinatorial power, language would become extremely cumbersome if it had to provide a separate name to differentiate every possible shape that might be visible in something as mundane as this patch of soil, and, moreover, to specify its exact location with the fine precision required here. However, the work of adequately locating and characterising relevant phenomena in the surround can be readily accomplished within talk-in-interaction if sign systems containing different kinds or resources for constituting phenomena, such as language and symbiotic gestures, are used in conjunction with each other.

Saussure (1959: 16) called for a science focused on the general study of signs. However, like most work in Semiotics that followed, he then defined his task as the study of a single semiotic system, in his case language. The study of how individual semiotic systems are organised has made enormous contributions to our understanding of the cognitive and social organisation of humans and of other animals. However, as the data being examined here demonstrate, it is also necessary to investigate how different sign systems work together to build relevant action and accomplish consequential meaning. By virtue of this potential synergy (indeed symbiotic relationships between systems of signs) any single system need provide only a partial specification of what is necessary to accomplish relevant meaning and action. Thus in both lines 7 and 21 the talk alone is not sufficient to specify what is being requested. Neither could the gestures that occur stand by themselves without the talk that accompanies them. Talk and gesture are further elaborated by the orientation displays and participation frameworks being constituted through other aspects of the participants' embodied conduct. And, again, none of these systems in isolation would be sufficient to construct the actions that the participants are pursuing. This suggests the importance of not focusing analysis exclusively on the properties of individual sign systems, but instead investigating the organisation of the ecology of sign systems which have evolved in conjunction with each other within the primordial site for human action: multiple participants using talk to build action while attending to the distinctive properties of a relevant setting.

The term ecology is used to note the way in which these separate systems function as differentiated, interdependent components of a larger whole that can adapt to changing circumstances. For example, in other research (Goodwin, 1995, 2000b) I have investigated how a man with severe aphasia (he can say only three words) is nonetheless able to act as an effective participant in conversation. This ability is not something lodged within him as an isolated individual, but instead is made possible through the way in which he and his interlocutors reorganise the sign systems used to construct meaning and action within interaction. For example, a single individual, the speaker, typically produces both talk and the gestures that accompany that talk (for example, all of the data examined here). Since the man with aphasia can't speak he produces gestures, while his co-participants provide the talk explicating the gesture, frequently in the form of guesses as to what he wants to say through the gesture. The basic symbiotic structure in which gesture gets its locally relevant sense from the way in which it both is elaborated by, and elaborates the talk that accompanies it remains intact. However, to adapt to one party's catastrophic loss of one of these sign systems, there is a rearrangement of the parties responsible for producing different kinds of signs. In short, there is a reorganisation of the contextual environment, the ecology tying separate sign systems to each other, which provides for the intelligibility of his gesture.

From a slightly different perspective, the way in which the structure of gesture differs markedly from language might reflect not the development of a new, more complex, system from a simpler one, but instead a process of progressive differentiation within a larger set of interacting systems in which gesture is organised precisely to provide participants with resources that complement, and thus differ significantly from, those afforded by language. Some support for the argument is provided by research (Bloom, 1979; Goldin-Meadow *et al.*, 1996; McNeill, 1992) in which fully competent speakers are asked to communicate while remaining silent. Under such circumstances their gestures quickly become more conventionalised, and linked into patterned sequences showing evidence of grammaticalisation. More generally the deictic expressions that are conventionalised in language, such as the 'this' that points toward the symbiotic gesture in line 7 (and the 'there' in line 19, and so on), constitute systematic ways of providing explicit links between different kinds of sign systems that characteristically function as parts of a larger whole.

In short, when one looks closely at how action is built within actual human interaction one frequently finds a cluster of quite different kinds of sign systems, for example talk and gesture lodged within a focus of visual and cognitive orientation constituted through embodied participation frameworks, and unfolding sequential organisation. Moreover, what is being focused on in the surround may itself have meaningful structure that can be used by participants as a resource for the construction of relevant action (Goodwin, 2000a). It would seem that something like this set of concurrently relevant semiotic fields is what is being pointed at by the phrase 'face-to-face interaction'. However, this is by no means a fixed array of fields. Thus on many occasions, such as phone calls, or when participants are dispersed in a large visually inaccessible environment (for example a hunting party, or a workgroup interaction through computers), visible co-orientation may not be present, and action might be built largely through talk alone, or through writing and images (Goodwin and Goodwin, 1996). Again, the set of mutually interacting sign systems used to build action functions as a dynamic ecology that can change to adapt to modifications in local circumstances.

Embodiment as public practice

Sue is faced with the task of learning to see as an archaeologist. Vision is usually analysed as a psychological process, as something done in the neurological or mental life of an individual. However, an analysis of vision that treats it as a purely psychological process, and especially one that sees vision as something lodged within the private mental life of the individual runs into serious problems here. To be a competent archaeologist Sue must be able to see archaeological features in the soil, to excavate them in a way that reveals their relevant structure, and to transform them into the documents, categories and maps that animate the life of her profession. The question posed for archaeology, indeed for any profession, is how such professional vision (Goodwin, 1994) can be systematically organised, such that others can trust her to competently see what should be seen in a patch of soil, and rely upon the maps and reports she makes. In short, how can vision be organised as public practice lodged within the worklife of a community?

The activities which have been investigated here constitute one solution to this problem. Shared orientation both to each other, and relevant phenomena in the environment (for instance the soil being excavated) is publicly established when participants use their bodies to create participation frameworks. The phenomena being scrutinised are constituted as meaningful entities through the talk in progress, the activity that talk is embedded within, and the emerging sequential organisation. Moreover, these same practices can be used to assess the actions being performed by each other's bodies (for example to note Sue's failure to do something that has been requested, to judge the accuracy of a line her hand is making, and so on). Within this domain of meaningful public scrutiny symbiotic gestures link the materials that are the focus of archaeological work, the soil being excavated, to the work being done by the participants' hands to locate and prepare for mapping relevant phenomena. Moreover, by virtue of the public character of this embodied work individual differences in how something should be seen can be negotiated. In data not examined here (Goodwin, in press) after Sue draws an outline, Ann uses her finger to

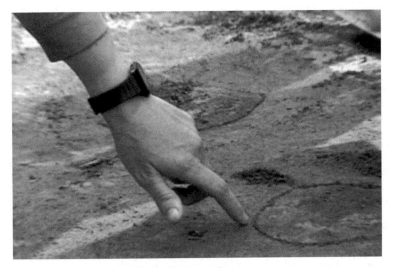

Figure 2.10

draw another line alongside Sue's; Ann thus shows Sue where she would have located the feature (see Figure 2.10).

The way in which symbiotic gestures annotate relevant phenomena within a public visual field provides participants with the resources necessary for systematically calibrating their practices of seeing. Moreover, in so far as this vision is made public through work and gesture, the entrainment of Sue's body into the demands of her profession extends beyond vision to encompass the full suite of embodied practices (using her trowel to reveal structure in the soil, shading the area being worked on with her body so that structures can be easily seen, linking what is visible to relevant categories, and so on) required to competently do the work of excavation.

In brief, the ecology of sign systems articulated through the work that defines a profession structures embodiment in human interaction as a way of knowing and shaping in detail a consequential world in concert with others.

Notes

1. A topic in gesture research that is relevant to what is being examined here is Pointing. This was the subject of a recent Max Planck conference organised by Sotaro Kita (Kita, in press). Analysis draws upon both the psychological and the interactive traditions. Pointing is certainly not only relevant to, but an element of, the symbiotic gesture in example 1. However, in much

investigation of pointing, objects in the surround are not analysed as components of the gesture itself. Instead, what is pointed at is treated as something outside the gesture, for example the target of a point. Moreover, not all symbiotic gestures are accomplished through pointing. In brief, while pointing is most relevant to what is being investigated here, it is a slightly different phenomenon.

2. See Lynch (1988) for analysis of how scientists progressively refine the images they are working with.

References

Bateson, Gregory (1972) *Steps to an Ecology of Mind*. New York: Ballantine Books.

Bloom, Ralph (1979) 'Language Creation in the Manual Modality: A Preliminary Investigation'. Bachelor's thesis, University of Chicago.

Damasio, Antonio (1994) *Descartes' Error: Emotion Reason, and the Human Brain*. New York: Grosset/ G.P. Putnam's Sons.

Damasio, Antonio (1999) *The Feeling of What Happens: Body and Emotion in the Making of Consciousness*. New York, San Diego, London: Harcourt Brace & Company.

Goffman, Erving (1964) 'The Neglected Situation'. In John J. Gumperz and Dell Hymes (eds)*The Ethnography of Communication*. American Anthropologist 66, 6, pt. II, 133–6.

Goldin-Meadow, Susan, McNeill, David, and Singleton, Jenny (1996) 'Silence is Liberating – Removing the Handcuffs on Grammatical Expression in the Manual Modality'. *Psychological Review* 103(1): 34–55.

Goodwin, Charles (1981) *Conversational Organization: Interaction Between Speakers and Hearers*. New York: Academic Press.

Goodwin, Charles (1986) 'Gesture as a Resource for the Organization of Mutual Orientation'. *Semiotica* 62(1/2): 29–49.

Goodwin, Charles (1987) 'Forgetfulness as an Interactive Resource'. *Social Psychology Quarterly* 50, No.2: 115–30.

Goodwin, Charles (1994) 'Professional Vision'. *American Anthropologist* 96(3): 606–33.

Goodwin, Charles (1995) 'Co-constructing Meaning in Conversations with an Aphasic Man'. *Research on Language and Social Interaction* 28(3): 233–60.

Goodwin, Charles (2000a) 'Action and Embodiment Within Situated Human Interaction'. *Journal of Pragmatics* 32(1489–1522).

Goodwin, Charles (2000b) Gesture, Aphasia and Interaction. In D. McNeill (ed.) *Language and Gesture*. Cambridge: Cambridge University Press, 84–98.

Goodwin, Charles (2002) 'Time in Action'. *Current Anthropology* 43.

Goodwin, Charles (in press) 'Pointing as Situated Practice'. In S. Kita (ed.) *Pointing: Where Language, Culture and Cognition Meet*. Hillsdale, NJ: Lawrence Erlbaum Associates.

Goodwin, Charles, and Goodwin, Marjorie Harness (1996) 'Seeing as a Situated Activity: Formulating Planes'. In Y. Engeström and D. Middleton (eds) *Cognition and Communication at Work*. Cambridge: Cambridge University Press, 61–95.

Goodwin, Marjorie Harness (1997) 'By-Play: Negotiating Evaluation in Story-telling'. In G.R. Guy, C. Feagin, D. Schriffin and J. Baugh (eds) *Towards a*

Social Science of Language: Papers in Honor of William Labov 2: Social Interaction and Discourse Structures. Amsterdam/Philadelphia: John Benjamins, 77–102.

Goodwin, Marjorie Harness, and Goodwin Charles (1986) 'Gesture and Coparticipation in the Activity of Searching for a Word'. *Semiotica* 62(1/2): 51–75.

Haviland, John (1995) 'Mental Maps and Gesture Spaces: Land, Mind and Body in Two Contexts'. Paper delived at the Conference on Gesture Compared Cross-Linguistically, Linguistic Institute, University of New Mexico, July 7–10, 1995.

Haviland, John (1998) 'Early Pointing Gestures in Zincantán'. *Journal of Linguistic Anthropology* 8(2): 162–96.

Haviland, John B. (1996) 'Projections, Transpositions, and Relativity'. In J.J. Gumperz and S.C. Levinson (eds) *Rethinking Linguistic Relativity*. Cambridge: Cambridge University Press, 271–323.

Heath, Christian (1986) *Body Movement and Speech in Medical Interaction*. Cambridge: Cambridge University Press.

Heath, Christian, and Hindmarsh Jon (2000) 'Configuring Action in Objects: From Mutual Space to Media Space'. *Mind, Culture and Activity* 7(1&2): 81–104.

Heath, Christian, and Luff Paul (1996) 'Convergent Activities: Line Control and Passenger Information on the London Underground'. In Y. Engeström and D. Middleton (eds) *Cognition and Communication at Work*. Cambridge: Cambridge University Press, 96–129.

Hindmarsh, Jon, and Heath, Christian (2000) 'Embodied Reference: A Study of Deixis in Workplace Interaction'. *Journal of Pragmatics*. 32, 12, 1855–78.

Hutchins, Edwin, and Palen, Leysia (1997) 'Constructing Meaning from Space, Gesture, and Speech'. In L. Resnick, R. Säljö, C. Pontecorvo and B. Burge (eds) *Discourse, Tools and Reasoning: Essays on Situated Cognition*. Springer-Verlag, 23–40.

Jefferson, Gail (1974) 'Error Correction as an Interactional Resource'. *Language in Society* 2: 181–99.

Johnson, Mark (1987) *The Body in the Mind: The Bodily Basis of Meaning, Imagination, and Reason*. Chicago: University of Chicago Press.

Kendon, Adam (1980) 'Gesture and Speech: Two Aspects of the Process of Utterance'. In M.R. Key (ed) *Nonverbal Communication and Language*. The Hague: Mouton, 207–77.

Kendon, Adam (1986) 'Some Reasons for Studying Gesture'. *Semiotica* 62: 3–28.

Kendon, Adam (1990a) *Conducting Interaction: Patterns of Behavior in Focused Encounters*. Cambridge: Cambridge University Press.

Kendon, Adam (1990b) Spatial Organization in Social Encounters: The F-Formation System. In A. Kendon (ed.) *Conducting Interaction: Patterns of Behavior in Focused Encounters*. Cambridge: Cambridge University Press, 209–38.

Kendon, Adam (1995) 'Gestures as Illocutionary and Discourse Structure Markers in Southern Italian Conversation'. *Journal of Pragmatics* 23: 247–79.

Kendon, Adam (1997) 'Gesture'. *Annual Review of Anthropology* 26: 109–28.

Kita, Sotaro (ed.) (in press) *Pointing: Where Language, Culture and Cognition Meet*. Hillsdale, NJ: Lawrence Erlbaum.

Krauss, R.M., Morrel-Samuels, P., and Colasante, C. (1991) 'Do Conversational Gestures Communicate?' *Journal of Personality and Social Psychology* 61: 743–54.

Lakoff, George, and Johnson, Mark (1999) *Philosophy in the Flesh: the Embodied Mind and its Challenge to Western Thought.* New York: Basic Books.

LeBaron, Curtis (1998) 'Building Communication: Architectural Gestures and the Embodiment of Ideas'. Ph. D dissertation, Department of Communition, The University of Texas at Austin.

LeBaron, Curtis D., and Streeck, Jürgen (2000) 'Gestures, Knowledge, and the World'. In D. McNeill (ed.) Gestures in Action, Language, and Culture. Cambridge: Cambridge University Press, pp. 118–38.

Lynch, Michael (1988) 'The Externalized Retina: Selection and Mathematization in the Visual Documentation of Objects in the Life Sciences'. *Human Studies* 11: 201–34.

McNeill, David (1992) *Hand & Mind: What Gestures Reveal About Thought.* Chicago: University of Chicago Press.

Nevile, Maurice (2001) 'Beyond the Black Box: Talk-in-Interaction in the Airline Cockpit'. Ph.D dissertation, Department of Linguistics, Australian National University.

Rimé, B, and Schiaratura, L. (1991) 'Gesture and Speech'. In R. Feldman and B. Rimé (eds) *Fundamentals of Nonverbal Behaviour.* Cambridge: Cambridge University Press. pp. 239–81.

Rizzolatti, Giacomo, and Arbib, Michael A. (1998) 'Language Within Our Grasp'. *Neuroscience* 21(5): 188–94.

Saussure, Ferdinand de (1959) *Course in General Linguistics.* Ed Charles Bally and Albert Sechehaye, in collaboration with Albert Riedlinger, translated from the French by Wade Baskin. New York: Philosophical Library.

Schegloff, Emanuel A. (1979) 'The Relevance of Repair for Syntax-for-Conversation'. In T. Givon (ed.) *Syntax and Semantics 12: Discourse and Syntax.* New York: Academic Press, pp. 261–88.

Schegloff, Emanuel A. (1984) 'On Some Gestures' Relation to Talk'. In J.M. Atkinson and J. Heritage (eds) *Structures of Social Action.* Cambridge: Cambridge University Press, pp. 266–96.

Schegloff, Emanuel A. (1992) 'Repair After Next Turn: The Last Structurally Provided Defense of intersubjectivity in Conversation'. *American Journal of Sociology* 97(5): 1295–345.

Schegloff, Emanuel A., Jefferson, Gail and Sacks, Harvey (1977) 'The Preference for Self-Correction in the Organization of Repair in Conversation'. *Language* 53: 361–82.

Streeck, Jürgen (1993) 'Gesture as Communication I: Its Coordination with Gaze and Speech'. *Communication Monographs* 60(4): 275–99.

Streeck, Jürgen (1994) 'Gestures as Communication II: The Audience as Co-Author'. *Research on Langauge and Social Interaction* 27(3): 223–38.

3

Transcending the Object in Embodied Interaction

Jon Hindmarsh and Christian Heath

Introduction

Despite a burgeoning body of studies concerned with the analysis of naturally occurring talk and discourse, relatively few augment their analyses with a consideration of the ways in which the body and material artefacts feature in, and work with, talk. In particular it is rather surprising to note that little analytic attention has been concerned with the ways in which talk and gesture combine over, around and with objects to produce meaningful discourse. For example, studies of discourse, particularly analyses of accounts of physical objects, rarely consider the ways in which the body enriches and elaborates talk about documents, paintings, tools, technologies and other aspects of material culture. In this chapter, we will explore how talk and embodied conduct is used to 'animate' or enliven physical objects in co-present interaction. Moreover, we will consider the ways in which individuals interweave talk and gesture over and around inanimate objects seemingly to infuse them with character and actions: character and actions that may otherwise remain unavailable.

To examine these embodied practices, we will provide examples from two everyday settings, classrooms and medical consultations, in which the participants are discussing quite distinct types of object. The section on university classrooms considers how students present works of craft for assessment. In particular we are concerned with the ways in which the students engage their bodies with inanimate objects to demonstrate how those objects, and sometimes an envisioned, yet-to-be-designed 'object', could or should be encountered, perceived or experienced by others. The section on medical consultations explores how gesture and other forms of bodily conduct are used to present suffering; to display, enact and (re)embody medical problems and difficulties. In this case, the body itself becomes the 'object' for animation. Despite the context-specific nature of the accounts, and indeed the objects, we would argue that these embodied practices are common to many routine activities in different ways. Thus, it is rather surprising that we have very little understanding of the character and interactional organisation of this embodied work with objects. Before discussing the analytical materials, it may be worth situating the relevance of the analysis for two distinct bodies of literature: non-verbal communication and the emerging sociology of the object.

Background

It is widely recognised that an attention to visual conduct as well as talk in studies of face-to-face interaction can enrich analytic purchase on the character and range of activities in which the participants are engaged. It has been powerfully argued, for example, that the ways in which people organise turns at talk does not solely rely upon vocal practices and resources, but can equally be influenced by gaze and gesture (see Goodwin, 1981). Despite the rich and varied body of work concerned with how talk and gesture are interrelated, indeed how they should be treated as a 'partnership' (Kendon, 2000), there is little consideration of the ways in which talk and gestures are figured with regard to the local ecology of objects. As Goodwin and Goodwin note, it is as if 'work on gesture in interaction (and deixis in linguistics) has drawn a bubble around the perimeters of the participants' bodies. The body of the actor has not been connected to the built world within which it is situated' (Goodwin and Goodwin, 1992: 37). Indeed, within the traditional linguistic literatures, even studies of demonstrative reference pay scant attention to the physical act of pointing, let alone the material artefacts through and to which the gesture passes (Hindmarsh and Heath, 2000).

Nevertheless, there is a growing body of work concerned with the ways in which the partnership of talk and gesture figures, and is figured by, the material ecology (see, for example, Goodwin, 1995; Goodwin, 1998; Goodwin, this volume; Heath and Luff, 2000; Hindmarsh and Heath, 2000; Streeck, 1996; Wootton, 1994). One reason for this interest in talk, gesture and the local ecology is the analytic commitment of such studies to understanding interaction in naturalistic settings; that is, to consider how participants produce and encounter embodied conduct in everyday, rather than lab-based, conditions. Such a commitment encourages the analyst to consider the contexts of particular relevance to the participants in face-to-face interaction themselves. One of those contexts is the material surround in and through which interaction is organised and accomplished. Such a concern is critical if we are to understand the organisation of gesture in interaction, for as LeBaron and Streeck put it, 'Without the index of the world of things, the movement of the hand could not be seen as an action, and the signifier would be lost in a sea of meaningless motion' (LeBaron and Streeck, 2000: 119). So later, when we turn to examples of interaction from education and medicine, we will consider how aspects of the local ecology are incorporated into the partnership of talk and gesture. Moreover, we will discuss the relevance of considering objects for understanding the very activities in which the participants are engaged.

Whilst the chapter is concerned to demonstrate the importance of analysing gestures in the material, and social interactional, realm in which they are produced and understood, the issues also bear upon a quite different body of research that might loosely be termed a 'sociology of the object'. Despite the pervasiveness of objects in everyday life, be they physical artefacts, digital representations or images, they have not, until relatively recently, received a great deal of attention within the social sciences. Indeed, social science has developed a curiously 'dis-embedded' characterisation of human conduct and sociality (see Heath and Hindmarsh, 2000; Heath and Hindmarsh, 2000). There are, of course, important exceptions, for example the writings of Marx, particularly the early manuscripts where he discusses praxis and action and the ways in which objects consist of congealed human activity (Marx, 1977). Or in a very different manner, consider Mead's discussion of the interdependence of the 'organism and the environment' and the relationship between artefacts and practical action (Mead, 1934). However, *empirical* studies of how objects and sociality intertwine have, until recently, been relatively rare.

It is perhaps in the work of Latour that we find some of the most vehement contemporary arguments for the (re)instatement of the object in sociology (see, for example, Latour, 1992). And subsequent empirical studies in Actor-Network Theory (ANT) and within the sociology of scientific knowledge have perhaps had the most profound impact on our understanding of objects and artefacts. However, the growing body of research concerned with the object is by no means limited to Actor-Network Theory. Social constructionism, symbolic interactionism, situated and distributed cognition, activity theory and ethnomethodology have all in different ways informed a diverse range of studies which (re)configure the relationship between social action and material realities. These studies and the diverse perspectives they embody criss-cross a range of substantive and disciplinary boundaries, from semiotics to sociology, from cognitive science to anthropology. Nevertheless, and despite the substantial contributions of this growing body of work, there remains relatively little research concerned with the ways in which objects feature in specific courses of action and interaction. So, for example, how individuals notice, invoke, refer to, examine, assess, discuss, even simply look at objects, both alone and together, remains under-explored.

So, although the idea that objects in our environment have a fundamentally interdependent relationship with social organisation is not new to the human sciences, there has been very little empirical research on the ways in which objects feature in specific courses of action and interaction. As a result, we have relatively little understanding of *how* objects enter into and are interconnected with social organisation, and indeed how they feature in practical activities, such as collaborative work (see Hindmarsh and Heath, 2000).

In this chapter, we will consider how objects are not simply referred to, but rather how they are drawn into embodied discourse: discourse concerned either with the objects themselves or indeed other (real or imagined) objects. We will see how individuals infuse their bodies with properties of objects; how individuals are able to produce for the here and now envisioned, previously experienced or otherwise unavailable characteristics of objects. Thus, in exploring the details of interaction, we aim to explicate the ways in which objects are brought into social action and interaction and how those objects can switch between the topic and the resource for embodied conduct.

To explore action and interaction with and around objects, we will refer to audio-visual materials collected by the researchers. We consider such recordings to be a powerful analytic resource, especially given the tacit and fleeting nature of the kinds of phenomena under scrutiny. Recorded materials provide the analyst with repeated access to the details and contingencies of their production. In this way, although video provides only one version of (or perspective on) events, it provides a continuously available resource. Thus, video allows us to draw together a concern with both the verbal and non-vocal elements of collaborative work and to analyse the ways in which these different elements of conduct are interwoven in action and interaction.

Intriguingly video rarely serves as an analytic resource in the social sciences and we have argued elsewhere that this derives from the lack of many methodological orientations able to handle such materials (see Heath and Hindmarsh, in 2000). Our methodological approach has similarities with a number of video-based interactional studies that draw on the writings of Harold Garfinkel, Harvey Sacks, Erving Goffman, Adam Kendon and others (for example, Goodwin, 1981; Goodwin, 1994, Goodwin, 1995; Heath, 1986; Heath and Luff, 2000; Wootton, 1994; and in a different vein Streeck, 1996; LeBaron and Streeck, 2000). This emerging tradition of interaction analysis inter-leaves field observations with the detailed analysis of video data. A fundamental analytic resource for this type of work is the moment-to-moment sequential organisation of interaction in which each action is both context shaped and context renewing, both organised in the light of the prior and framing the next (Heritage, 1984). It provides us with the resources to unpack the ways in which interaction is produced, managed and unfolds *in situ* (for a recent methodological discussion, see Heath and Hindmarsh, 2000).

Gesturing craft

The first research domain features university craft and design students presenting their work to peers and tutors for evaluation. Although we will discuss only a few fragments of action and interaction, these are situated within fairly lengthy sessions in which four or five students present their work. These sessions, the activities and the objects involved, have some notable features relevant to the ways in which the works of craft are presented and discussed. First, there is a range of different kinds of object discussed within the course of these presentations. The work consists not of the 'final' object, as it might for an essay, but rather of a variety of objects that reveal the work at various stages in the development of their project. Thus, students narrate their project work with reference to preliminary sketches and drawings, through to models and (constituent parts of) the (nearly complete) articles. Before each session the students assemble their objects in the parts of the room from which they will present. Secondly, the tutors continually encourage their students to look beyond the current state of their work to consider where their artefact should be deployed, how it could be presented and how they would like the object to be used, seen, encountered or experienced. Thus, the students often refer to particular categories of (intended) user, for example 'businessmen', 'designers', 'young people', 'my mates', and so on. Therefore, many of the discussions of the objects relate to envisioned futures for the artefacts, rather than their status in the here and now.

A practical problem for the students, then, is how to present the current (often unfinished) objects in such a way as to give a sense of the envisioned future for the object and the people who will use or encounter it. We want to show how the embodied conduct of the students over, around and with their craft work overcomes this practical problem. These practices enable the students to present: envisioned places in which their objects could be encountered; uses and activities in which they would feature; and perspectives from which users would experience them.

To give a flavour of these issues, consider the first data fragment which features Oliver,[1] who was instructed to produce something using rubber as one of its main components. In undertaking the task, he has begun to develop a new type of briefcase designed for people who need to keep documents flat whilst they travel from place to place. His design uses two flat pieces of wood pulled tightly together by taut rubber. To enhance the mobility of the briefcase he intends to mount it on wheels. However, the actual work is at a very early stage. He has cut the wood, but not been successful in attaching the rubber. As his commentary begins in Fragment 3.1, he is referring to a diagram of the concept that he has drawn on to a piece of card. He explains what the briefcase would look like before going on to discuss how it would be used. The fragments are transcribed using the orthography developed by Gail Jefferson (see Jefferson, 1984).[2]

Fragment 3.1

O: >I came up with an idea which is that.< (1.0)
It's: erm: (.) like a <u>sol</u>id wooden <u>ba</u>se (.) and rear. (.) and
it's got- it's like (.) corrugated in rubber down the sides.
so that erm, (.) you can stre::tch it, you can like pull it
open. if >say it'd be this sort of shape< you can pull it open
and put stuff in it right down. (.)
<u>file</u>:s and and erm, (0.8) notes and stuff.
and it's like a briefcase sort of thing (.)
and erm because it's in rubber you can basically keep
stretching it as far as far as you want.
so you can put loads and loads of stuff in it.

At the onset of the fragment, Oliver is running his finger over the lines already drawn on the card. These lines feature in his sketch of the brief-case and he is referring to them to highlight the elements of the briefcase that he is describing, namely the 'solid wooden base (.) and rear' and the corrugated rubber that runs down the sides (see Figure 3.1, Picture Pair a). Having discussed the features depicted on the card, he then begins to use the card in quite a different way. Rather than refer to features on it, he incorporates it into a mime about how someone would use the finished briefcase.

In fact, he uses the card to act as a proxy for one side of the envi-sioned object. He does this first by producing a stretching gesture away from the card as if taking hold of the other envisioned wooden surface and pulling it away from the card he has in his hand. Then he turns the card around to give a sense of the orientation of the envisioned briefcase, whilst he says 'say it'd be this sort of shape'. By changing the orientation of the card Oliver reveals how the object would stand in relation to the body. Again he begins to demonstrate how someone would open up the briefcase (see Figure 3.1, Picture Pair b). Finally he displays how documents would be inserted into the briefcase, using his flattened hand no longer to 'hold' one side of the briefcase, but rather to symbolise a document (see Figure 3.1, Picture Pair c).

Thus, Oliver incorporates the card into what Kendon calls a 'gesticu-lation' (discussed in Kendon, 1982). An example of a gesticulation is when a person says 'and then she pulled back the lever' whilst grab-bing an imaginary lever and producing a pulling motion back towards the body. Here, however, we encounter what might be termed an 'object-centred gesticulation', that incorporates a physical object into the production of the gesture. This gesticulation is produced with the piece of card as a critical component. Moreover, Oliver uses the card that he has at hand to stand on behalf of a part of the envisioned brief-case rather than the actual wooden surfaces that lie a hand's reach away. Thus, we can see how the physical card with the concept drawing on it switches from being the explicit *topic* of the talk to being an interactional *resource* for animating the envisioned briefcase.

A sense of the object as part of an envisioned whole is achieved only when the gestures over, around and with the card are analysed as they are produced and encountered – in real-time sequential order. Oliver builds up the sense of the envisioned object through the juxtaposition of one gesture with the next, and with one part of the verbal descrip-tion and the next. The movement from referencing the diagram on the card to miming with the card is achieved through the partnership of

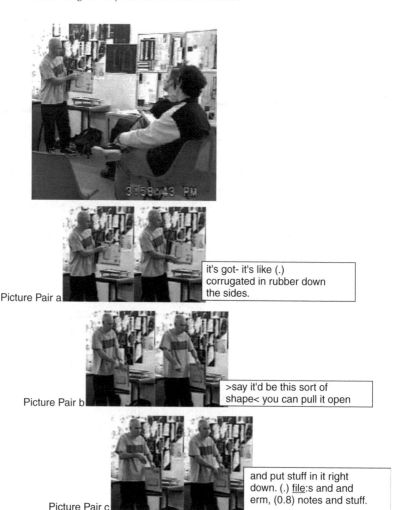

Picture Pair a

it's got- it's like (.) corrugated in rubber down the sides.

Picture Pair b

>say it'd be this sort of shape< you can pull it open

Picture Pair c

and put stuff in it right down. (.) file:s and and erm, (0.8) notes and stuff.

Figure 3.1   Images for Fragment 3.1

talk and embodied conduct. He does not explicitly say 'as you can see here' but rather talks purely about the envisioned object (represented by drawing or gesticulation) whilst altering his body's visible relation to the card – pointing at features of it, then making a pulling motion alongside it. Only through seeing the changing orientation of the card to the gestures and the body around it do we get a sense of its use and relevance. Oliver succeeds in creating the scene in which the envisioned use of a not-yet-produced briefcase is recognisably acted out.

Not only does Oliver gesticulate the act of opening the briefcase and the direction and angle of opening, but also his bodily performance reveals a sense of the quality of the experience of opening the envisioned briefcase. He manages to perform the very *resistance* associated with opening the briefcase, a resistance attributable to the corrugated rubber. Intriguingly he makes no reference whatsoever to this quality in his talk, but nevertheless provides a sense of it through the way he mimes – almost as intonation accentuates utterances, here the character of the gesticulation gives a sense of the rubber's resistance. This resistance or tension is embodied in the gesticulation through the ways in which Oliver tenses and stiffens his arms, raises his shoulders and how his left hand noticeably grips the physical card harder. Each of these fairly minor changes work together to give a sense of strain and effort, an effort clearly not imposed by the action is which he is engaged, as he is pulling at thin air. Nevertheless, he manages to perform resistance and thereby create an impression of the strength of an invisible rubber.

Later, as he says 'keep stretching it as far as you want', he does not 'open' the envisioned case in one smooth movement, but rather charts the resistance through multiple smaller movements or 'yanks'. He even throws his head back slightly which gives a suggestion of the effort and tension involved. So, in a way we're starting to see how the *material qualities* of the envisioned object are made available for the audience, material qualities that are not readily available through the objects alone.

Paterson has argued that particular works of art, most notably sculptures, provide a sense of what it would be like to touch them; they give the promise of tactility, even if touching is not a real possibility (Paterson, in preparation). Thus Paterson argues that such objects, maybe all objects, have a tactile 'investment' in space. Here the student designer in the first example is attempting to demonstrate the tactile properties of (aspects of) the briefcase he is designing. However, these properties are not made available by the objects on show but rather *he* invests a resistance and tension in space through his gestures and through his bodily conduct. By taking the role of the envisioned user, he brings to life the materials, and relevant properties of the materials, that would constitute the briefcase. Moreover, his performance places himself in the role of the user and the audience as witnessing his use of the briefcase.

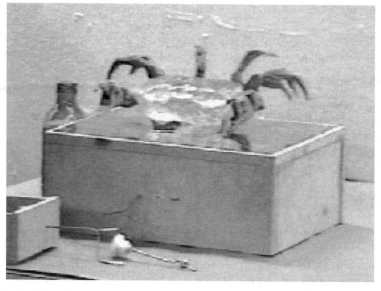

Figure 3.2 Alan's crab

However, the student designers do not always take the role of a possible user of one of their designed objects, but rather can infuse their bodies with properties of the object itself. Take, for example, Fragment 3.2, in which Alan is presenting a near-complete work. He has taken on the challenge of designing an automata; that is a craftwork that has some dynamic properties to be triggered by external stimulus, usually an individual pressing a button, rolling a wheel or whatever. In this case, Alan has produced a 'crab' (see Figure 3.2).

He filled the shell of a real crab with resin in order to produce the body. Then, he carved wooden legs and pincers which he attached to the resin body. Finally, he mounted the finished crab on to a copper-plated wooden box and attached wires from the crab's legs and pincers to a crank hidden inside the box. When someone turns the crank, the legs move up and down and make a rather unnerving tapping sound on the copper plate. In addition, the pincers slowly and menacingly open and close. As the fragment begins, Alan and the tutor are considering the most appropriate way of displaying the crab and how different ways of mounting it could highlight different properties – both visual and aural.

Fragment 3.2

T: Maybe you could have it at- sort of a- slight <u>ang</u>:le or
    some:thing?=
A: =May:be, but I quite li:ke the idea of er: (.) these claws
    <u>snappin</u>' at ya.=
S: =hhhumh.=
A: =Facin you, you know.=
T: =[<u>Yes</u>:. yes.=
S: [hmmm
A: =And sort of <u>sat</u> <u>back</u> (.) and he's <u>aim</u>ing 'em at whoevers
    turning the handle.

In the course of arguing that the crab should lie flat rather than be
tilted, Alan demonstrates how he would like the crab to be encountered. As he says 'these claws <u>snappin</u>' at ya', he points at the crab's
claws and then uses both of his hands to make a snapping motion at
the tutor. In doing this, the snapping claws of the crab are disam-
biguated from the range of crab movements, such as the legs tapping
and so forth. Alan mimes some of the actions of the crab by snapping
his fingers together, pincer-like, as he rears up to face the tutor. This
mime exaggerates particular features of the crab relevant to his case
and withholds others. Maintenance of the coherence of the crab's relationship to the body of the student is accomplished in various ways.
First, Alan points to the claws whilst looking at them, thereby drawing
the gaze of others to the crab's claws. Also he rears up and turns
directly at the tutor as the actions of the claws are transposed into his
body and directed outwards. Even following this initial demonstration,
he turns back to the crab and turns the handle to show the claws snapping, dropping his arm low to allow people to see it. By repeatedly
drawing attention alternately to the crab and his own actions, Alan
maintains their juxtaposition.

In part, the transposition of the action to the body provides a particular perspective for the viewer – a perspective that has local relevance
but also transcends the local as it deals with how another may
encounter the crab in the future. The body is used as a proxy for the
object such that a sense of how the object should be experienced is
made available to the audience. Whereas in Fragment 3.1 the student
momentarily took the place of a user of the envisioned briefcase, here
Alan infuses his body with particular properties of the crab itself in

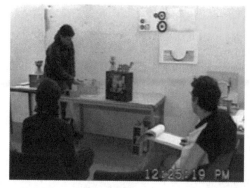

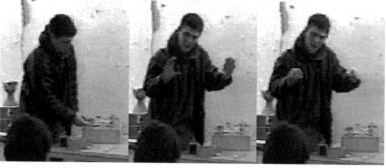

Figure 3.3   Images for Fragment 3.2

order to place the audience (notably, but not solely, the tutor) in the role of a user. He provides the audience with a particular perspective on the crab that an envisioned user would ideally be confronted with. He presents the claws of the crab opening and closing as the crank is turned. His body allows him to enlarge the scale and impact of the key crab actions and disambiguate those actions from a range of other visual and aural effects. Thus, the body is used to conjure up a large scale 'crab' to confront and 'snap at' the audience.

He actually produces the full demonstration twice. First, during 'snappin' at ya'. Then there is a slight pause before he produces it again during 'Facin' you, you know'. Alan is looking at the tutor throughout and just at the moment the tutor starts to display his understanding 'Yes:. yes.', Alan's hands drop and the mime is finished. Thus the mime is recycled and continues until some appreciation of the sense and relevance of the mime is forthcoming. In such a way, the mime can be seen to be designed and emerge with regard to the visible and vocal participation and involvement of the tutor. They are discussing a particular design decision regarding how to display the crab to maximise its impact. The mime works beautifully to enliven a particular property of the crab, a particular perspective on the menacing moving claws, and to encourage the tutor to align with the impact of that property and thus a particular way of displaying the crab.

So, the students use their talk and bodily conduct to produce an image for the local audience of someone using the unfinished wooden briefcase and also to put the local audience in the position of encountering a large-scale version of the crab snapping in action. The craft work, then, is not described in isolation, but is related to the uses and activities in which the work could be encountered and explored. Even the aesthetic value of the crab is demonstrated through its placement in a vision of how it would be encountered and what a user would be confronted by.

Here we see these student designers actually giving figure to, forming, bringing into shape and life the envisioned users of their designs and their potential or idealised activities with, or perspectives on, those designs. These practices we see as produced through both talk and embodied conduct, each reflexively elaborating the other. Other studies of design have also noted how these embodied practices recurrently feature in the work of debating different design decisions (for example Büscher and Shapiro, 2000). They work as an aid to persuading others, showing others and enacting for others how particular designs could or would work when confronted by actual users. They work to present in the here and now, and for the local audience, envisioned futures for the designs-in-progress.

These embodied practices then are critical to the work of the designer and are one of the tacit practices associated with the design community. Whether in design meetings with clients, or in coursework evaluations, these practices help to give a sense of the trajectory of, and life to, the design-in-progress. As the crab example shows, such enactments also provide an opportunity for designers to highlight or emphasise the critical properties of particular designs, thereby demonstrating how it should be deployed or encountered. These are communications skills, skills of persuasion, that are not simply verbal, but employ a whole range of embodied conduct. This is not to argue that the embodied practices on show are skills available only to the designer. Indeed, they employ many mundane practices in order to engage in design work.

In different ways, therefore, we can begin to see how an artefact (a piece of card or a resin crab) can gain a sense and significance it might not otherwise have by virtue of the ways in which a participant may animate and manipulate it through their gesture and talk. The object becomes not so much part of the body as, rather, an integral feature of specific courses of action displayed by the body. Büscher has recently discussed the idea of imagination in action, considering how designers reason through successive formulations of objects (Büscher, 2001). Here we find a rather different aspect of imagination, namely the ways in which students, through their talk and bodily comportment, can provide co-participants with a sense of the potential significance of an object or design. Underlying this achievement are the ways in which the 'performance' is configured with regard to the perspective of 'someone' who might encounter and use the object within ordinary practical circumstances.

Re-embodying suffering

We would like to explore these issues a little further by considering one or two rather different instances; fragments in which the body itself becomes an object during medical encounters (see also Emerson, 1970; Heath, 1986; Hirschauer, 1991). The examples are drawn from the medical consultation and in particular from primary health care; a domain in which one of the authors holds a substantial corpus of data (see, for example, Heath, 1986; Heath, 1989; Heath and Luff, 2000; Greatbatch *et al.*, 1993). The general practice consultation is a rich and rewarding setting in which to consider how the body is configured within the course of particular activities. In the examples at hand we would like to adopt a rather different standpoint. Building on our earlier examples, we wish to briefly consider how the body itself becomes an 'object' with which a participant can reveal their experience and in this case suffering. It is, perhaps, worthwhile clarifying the issue more substantively.

The general practice consultation ordinarily begins with the patient providing their reason for seeking medical help or updating the doctor on the progress of their illness. In either case patients present and characterise their symptoms and suffering and the doctor initiates a series of inquiries to clarify certain characteristics of the difficulty. In some, but by no means all cases, patients actually show the difficulty to the doctor and its visible manifestation; a boil, a bruise, a rash, or whatever, temporarily becomes the principal visual focus and subject to inquiry and investigation. More often than not, however, there is no visible manifestation of the complaint. The patient has to provide the sense and significance of the illness and its symptoms through their talk and bodily conduct and thereby legitimise seeking the professional help of the doctor.

Consider the following example. It is drawn from the beginning of the consultation. The patient enters, sits down, and the doctor initiates the business at hand with 'what can we do for you'?

Fragment 3.3

    Dr: What can we do for you?
            (0.5)
    P: Well all weekend I've been getting these terrible
            headaches<it's:: (0.2) all sort of top of me head th<u>ere</u>::
            (.) an at the <u>back</u> (.) ˙hhh an when I get these
            headaches: if I move my eyes: from sort of side to side
            that (.) type of thing it really ach: (.) <u>a::ches</u> you know
            all (.) under me eyes: (.) ˙hhh on Sunday I noticed they
            went all <u>puffy</u> (0.2) a[n (red)
    Dr: [Yes
            (0.2)
    P: an I keep going <u>dizz</u>y (an) (0.5) you know hot and cold
            (.) it's a horrible feeling.

The patient's description of her difficulties is accompanied by a series of gestures: gestures that help reveal and give a sense of the particular character of each of her symptoms. She begins by locating the position of her headaches, not simply by describing and pointing to particular areas, but by clasping regions of her head. With her initial assessment, 'terrible headaches', the patient turns towards the doctor and begins to raise her hands to, and lowers, her head. As she utters the word 'it's' the hands clasp either side of her head. The pronoun, coupled with the arriving gesture, serves not simply to project more to follow (and secure the 'floor' for the patient) but neatly links the arriving gesture retrospectively to the 'terrible headaches' and prospectively to the upcoming characterisation. With the arriving hands, and 'it's', the doctor produces a slight reorientation and eyebrow raise, which nicely serves both to acknowledge the assessment and display continued alignment to the upcoming exposition. With 'it's all sort' the hands are

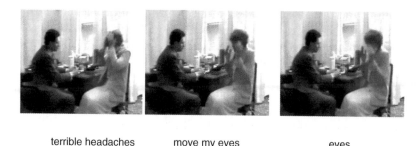

terrible headaches   move my eyes   eyes

Figure 3.4   Images for Fragment 3.3

slowly raised and firmly replaced in the same position; a moment later, with the word 'there', the hands are raised and clutch the back of the head. In touching and clasping the head, the hands are able to reveal more than simply the location and scope of the difficulty. Through the pace and pressure with which hands land on and hold the head, they provide, perhaps, a curious sense of both the tenderness of the head itself and the underlying pressure of the ache. This sense of the symptoms, however, is not simply embodied within the clasping, touching hands, but is prefigured in and reflexively constituted through the initial, spoken assessment 'terrible headaches' – the terrible captured beautifully in the hands' touching movements.

As the patient begins to describe the symptoms which arise with the headaches, she once more bodily animates her own bodily actions and sensation. As she continues with '·hhh an when' she removes her hands from her head and places them upright at either side of her head and eyes. With 'side to side' she enacts the action, turning her head from side to side whilst flapping her hands to visually exaggerate the direction of the movements. She then describes the symptom 'it really ach: (.) a::ches you know all (.) under me eyes:'. As she begins, she replaces her hands vertically alongside her eyes, and with 'it really' vibrates the hands as if the eyes are throbbing. A moment later, as she utters and repeats the word 'aches', elongating and emphasising the word the second time, she simulates a tenderness by appearing to carefully touch the area beneath her eyes, the fingers slowing almost to a halt as they near the skin. With and within the spoken description of the symptom, the hands and fingers not only foreshadow a description of the location of the difficulty, but provide a particular sense of the suffering. The vibrating fingers reveal the throbbing, intense character of the ache and the gentle, wary touch reveals the acute tenderness under the eyes. These gestures do not simply serve to illustrate the talk, but rather provide a particular flavour to the generalised description and embody characteristics of the illness not 'touched' on in the talk.

As she continues, the patient builds a series of further descriptions that rely upon various bodily activities to particularise and animate the character of the symptoms and suffering. The scope and intensity of the 'puffy red eyes', the 'dizziness' revealed through a vibrating head and falling forward, and 'hot and cold' with a flustered gesture. There is not space here to address these subsequent revelations; however, we can begin to see how the body itself can become the object for animation, which in turn is designed to reveal the characteristics and functioning of the body. Unlike the examples discussed in the first part of the chapter where action is related to works of craft, here the patient, through talk and bodily conduct, is animating and revealing aspects of the body, its functioning and their sensation.

Taking the symptoms and their respective locations in turn, the patient overlays particular parts of the body with a series of gestures. The gestures, with and within the talk, particularise and animate the symptoms; they give them a certain sense and significance and serve to reveal not just the symptom, but the symptom experienced by this patient. For example, the eyes do not simply ache when the head is moved from side to side, but they throb with pain and become acutely sensitive in the region below the eyes. The gestures demarcate the position, the scope and the character of the suffering. They *enliven*, if only momentarily, different parts of the body, and provide a dramatic display of the symptoms and suffering actually incurred by the patient. The gestures powerfully configure not just the symptoms, but the symptoms in action; they transform a description of the illness into a revelation of the difficulties experienced by the patient. The patient's bodily conduct embodies the symptoms suffered by the patient giving them a presence, a force, an existence, here and now, that they would not otherwise have.

Despite the absence of any physical manifestation of the complaint, the patient is able to demonstrate her symptoms to the doctor. She encourages the doctor, during the evolving course of the description, to align visually towards her and, at various moments, to look at and watch particular actions. The hands and fingers are juxtaposed, positioned and laid on or alongside parts of the body, and, with the talk, they transpose action to and within those bodily regions. The patient's gestures and bodily comportment serve to transform generic categories of complaint into unique and particular difficulties. Complaints such as sore throats, coughs, headaches and the like, which might even be thought rather trivial, are given a certain distinctiveness and significance that warrants medical intervention. They are revealed as difficulties that have entailed severe suffering by the patient. Thus patients particularise their problems through the ways in which they re-embody the experience of their symptoms.

We can begin to see how a patient can render their difficulties and their experience of their difficulties visible within the practical constraints of the medical consultation. Through talk, gesture and bodily conduct, patients transpose inner suffering, their personal subjective experience of their complaint, to the body's surface and particular parts and areas of their physique. The inner and the subjective is overlaid on the outer surface of the body and rendered visible and objective. Moreover, through visual, tactile and spoken conduct patients take symptoms experienced on another occasion and transpose them to the present. They reveal their symptoms, and their experience of their symptoms, here and now; revealing the very characteristics that they have been invited to describe. To use and slightly corrupt Wieder's (1974) phrase, patients render their symptoms 'transituational': transposing experience and conduct from one occasion to another. The doctor momentarily becomes a spectator: witness to the very symptoms that the patient has experienced or possibly is experiencing.

We can also begin to see how the gestures work with and within the talk, and, in particular, how they serve prospectively to display distinct qualities and the severity of the voiced symptom(s). The occurrence and articulation of these gestural embodiments can also be seen, in this brief sketch of the fragment, to be sensitive to, and relevant for, the participation of the doctor, and, in particular, the ways in which he should orient and respond to the characterisation. In other words, the patient's opportunity to display and re-embody their symptoms evolves within the developing course of the interaction with the doctor, and is dependent upon her ability to secure relevant forms of alignment and participation. We noted how, for example, in clasping her head and voicing the initial pronoun of her next utterance, the patient is not only able to secure the floor but project the upcoming relevance of a particular focal area and visual alignment for the co-participant. In turn, the doctor's acknowledgement and visual orientation provides the foundation for the bodily as well as spoken exposition of the problem. These gestures are designed and fashioned not simply with regard to some embodied display, but rather with regard to how that display can both secure the alignment of the recipient, and, in so doing, configure the revelation so as to maximise its visual impact on the other. Thus, as these gestures evolve, they are inextricably embedded within the emerging orientation and conduct of the co-participant.

We began by considering the ways in which the body and talk provide a vehicle to transpose action and characteristics to inanimate objects, to give them a sense and significance they might not otherwise have. We then considered how bodily conduct and talk can animate the self-same body to reveal symptoms and the individual's experience of those symptoms. In the final fragment, we wish to develop two aspects of these forms of activity; on the one hand the ways in which they involve and evolve a performance that is transposed and embedded within the object (in this case the body) and secondly their dependence upon the moment-by-moment co-participation of the (potential) recipient(s).

The following brief fragment (Fragment 3.4) is once again drawn from the beginning of a consultation. The patient is discussing the progress of his illness and its treatment. Following the doctor's query he mentions that he is still becoming tired when walking.

Fragment 3.4

Dr:	How are you do:in:?
	(0.8)
P:	Well I still get very <u>tir:ed:</u> (0.7) walking (.) <u>swe</u>at:.
	(0.8)
Dr:	Yeh
	(.)
P:	<u>phhewhhhhh</u>
	(1.0)
P:	I er:m::: (0.6) wrote down that er:: (0.4) sick place about that permanent retirement you know Doctor.

The patient's spoken reply appears relatively innocuous, simply mentioning one or two symptoms. It is accompanied, however, by a bodily performance in which symptoms are dramatically, yet subtly, revealed. With the word 'tired' the patient turns away from the doctor and shakes his head from side to side. It catches the doctor's eye and he turns from the medical record to watch the patient. The patient then looks down towards the floor, and once again shakes his head from

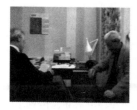 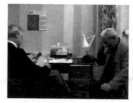 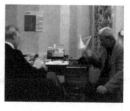

Well I still get very tir:ed   Walking (.) sweat:.   (0.2)

Figure 3.5   Images for Fragment 3.4

side to side. Coupled with the word 'tired' the patient's conduct appears to enact tiredness, the head shake and orientation revealing exhaustion, even, perhaps, dismay. The doctor provides no spoken or visible response. The patient begins to look up and takes the floor to speak, adding the word 'walking'. The word 'walking' recasts the sense of the bodily action and tiredness, respecifiying how the exhaustion derives from a particular kind of activity. Whilst watching the patient, the doctor remains unmoved; he produces neither visual nor vocal response and the performance passes without comment.

The patient then mentions an additional symptom, 'sweat'. With the word 'sweat' he looks down and mops his brow with his left hand even though there is no visible sweat lying upon the patient's face. He then looks at his open hand and seemingly inspects the imaginary sweat that he has removed from his brow. After a moment the patient lets his hand and arm fall on to the doctor's desk.

The doctor neither acknowledges the difficulties nor, as might ordinarily occur, does he initiate a series of further inquiries into the changing character of the illness. He appears to be looking at the patient but remains silent and unresponsive. As the brow is mopped the doctor turns to the medical records and a moment later produces 'yeh'. The shift in orientation, the engagement with the record, and the downward intoned 'yeh' provide little acknowledgement and certainly display no appreciation of the suffering apparently experienced by the patient.

The patient's actions do more than simply animate the parts of the body. They enact the very symptoms that the patient experiences when walking. His reorientation towards the floor, his slow lateral head shaking and the mopping of imaginary sweat reveal to the doctor, then and there within the occasion of the consultation, the symptoms that he suffers. The spoken description of symptoms provide a critical resource in recognising the character and significance of the bodily enactment, just as the bodily enactment gives substance to and particularises the voiced symptoms. Through his bodily conduct the patient illustrates, or, better, demonstrates, his symptoms, providing the doctor not just with an opportunity to hear of difficulties but to witness for himself the patient's suffering. The enactment takes the symptoms and displays not just the difficulties the patient suffers, but the patient's experience of the difficulties.

Like the other examples we have discussed in this chapter, it is difficult to discern how far the participant's demonstration achieves interactional significance. In the case at hand, the doctor provides little acknowledgement of either the symptoms or the patient's experiences. It would appear, however, that the patient's enactment is sensitive to the alignment and response, or absence of response, from the doctor. For example, the patient's reorientation towards the floor is prefigured and entails a series of lateral head movements, which successively secure a shift of orientation by the doctor from the records to the patient. The realignment of patient's gaze towards the doctor, coupled with the pause following the display of tiredness, might also be an attempt to secure some acknowledgement from the doctor. Moreover, the placing of the hand directly in front of the doctor and visually orienting to it might also be concerned not just with demonstrating the trouble but also with encouraging some greater display of appreciation and involvement (see Goodwin, 1981; Heath, 1986). It is also worthwhile mentioning that even following the doctor's minimal acknowledgement ('yeh') and his orientation back to the record, the patient does not necessarily abandon all attempts to have his symptoms and suffering addressed by the doctor. As the doctor utters 'yeh' and the patient places his elbow on the desk, he turns to one side, and exhales loudly, articulating through his breath '<u>phhewhhhhh</u>'. The character and sequential position of the loud exhalation suggests that it may not only serve to complete the revelation of the symptoms associated with walking, but perhaps encourage the doctor to provide further acknowledgement of the patient's difficulties.

The patient's description and demonstration of his difficulties does not occasion further inquiry or investigation from the doctor. They may, of course, be irrelevant, as far as the doctor is concerned, to the business at hand; which in turn raises an interesting question concerning the doctor's initial inquiry as to the patient's health, the discussion of symptoms and assessment in follow-up consultations (see Heath, 1992). Putting to one side the trouble that the patient takes to present and embody his difficulties and suffering, it is worth noting how the consultation in this case develops. Unusually, it is the patient, rather than the doctor, who initiates the next activity. On turning back to the doctor, who is still reading the records, the patient realigns the topic at hand from the symptoms and suffering to his attempt to deal with and manage the implications of his difficulties – to contact 'that sick place about permanent retirement'. In such a way the patient initiates what is sometimes characterised as the management phase of the consultation. This realignment of topic proves successful in that the doctor is quick to respond to and discuss how the matters in question might be handled. The patient's demonstration therefore appears to achieve neither interactional nor diagnostic significance, and simply becomes subsumed under the general management of a previously diagnosed complaint.

We can begin to see, therefore, how patients, within the practicalities of the medical consultation, attempt to provide the doctor with the sense and significance of their difficulties. The body becomes both the source of their difficulties and the vehicle through which they are portrayed and re-embodied. Through talk and bodily conduct patients transpose 'inner' experience and suffering to the surface of their body. They render their symptoms and suffering visible by undertaking a series of actions both with and overlaying their body; actions that transpose difficulties suffered on other occasions to the 'here and now'. These enactments and demonstrations provide patients with the possibility of presenting the unique and distinctive qualities of their illness and suffering. It is not, for example, *any* headache; it is a dramatic, intense, localised pain which renders the head highly sensitive; not any sore throat, but one which clasps the throat and chokes one; not any pain in the chest, but pain which momentarily overwhelms one, and so forth. In other words, enactment and demonstrations display the unique and particular qualities of pain and suffering; they give a distinctive sense and significance to generic categories of complaint and symptom.

Moreover, these revelations emerge in and through the patient's interaction with the doctor. To gain sense and significance, and sequential and diagnostic import, they require particular forms of co-participation from the (potential) recipient. In Fragment 3.3, like the examples discussed earlier in the chapter, we can see how the ways in which the gestured features of the activity are organised with regard to the visual orientation and alignment of the co-participant(s). For instance, the patient maintains her orientation towards the doctor, and animates features of her body, including her eyes and face, which are the principal focus of alignment of the doctor. The gestures themselves, such as the moving, framing hands for puffy eyes, may be simultaneously designed to display certain symptoms whilst preserving the relevant form of co-participation from the doctor. Unlike in Fragment 3.4, they succeed; the animated characteristics of the patient's symptoms are explicitly addressed by the doctor in the diagnosis (see Heath, forthcoming). In contrast, in Fragment 3.4 we can see how the patient's failure to establish a relevant form of co-participation from the doctor undermines the sequential significance of the enactment, and his bodily revelations of his suffering remain unexplored and unaddressed within the consultation. Moreover, we can see how the patient, in the course of producing his characterisation of his difficulties, builds the portrayal in the light of the doctor's seeming lack of alignment and in an attempt to secure relevant forms of co-participation from the recipient. The gestures discussed in the chapter emerge moment by moment in the light of the interaction between the co-participants, the displays, performances, revelations, and the like, products of evolving co-participation.

Discussion

The work of the young designers and the work of the patients discussed in this chapter have a common basis in the use of talk and embodied conduct to reveal in the here and now things that would otherwise remain hidden. Their work is critically not reducible to the discourse, or talk, that they use in the course of their activities, but rather relies upon the artful practices of embodied conduct. To develop a detailed understanding of the work of discussing designs or revealing symptoms, the analysis is enriched through examination of the visual as well as the vocal elements of that work. For these activities are truly embodied. The incorporation of physical objects into gesture and embodied conduct enables the participants to 'traverse' the visible and the imaginary: the past, present and envisioned futures of objects; indeed the material and the immaterial. Notions such as 'vision' or 'suffering' are often associated with 'inner', subjective experiences, but in these data we witness participants animating these phenomena and realising them in interaction with others. Thus, they exhibit embodied solutions to practical interactional problems for participants – to present a design vision or to demonstrate suffering. Moreover, the embodied solutions discussed here demonstrate how the ongoing talk, embodied conduct and the physical objects incorporated with them mutually elaborate one another. The sense and significance of each is only available in the context of the others.

Aside from contributing to our understanding of talk, gesture and embodied conduct, the materials also bear upon ways of understanding and analysing the 'agency' of objects. The contemporary concern with object (or more broadly, non-human) agency derives mainly from the programmatic commitment of Actor-Network Theory to 'radical symmetry': that is to accord humans and non-humans equivalent analytic status. This commitment has been realised in part through an attempt to analyse the agency not only of humans, but also non-humans in a network. These data, however, expose a rather different approach to the notion of agency. We see how participants themselves entail action in objects; they construe the envisioned or past agency of objects in and through their embodied conduct. In Fragment 3.2, for example, we are shown how the crab will be encountered 'snappin'' at the person turning the crank. In Fragment 3.3, on the other hand, a terrible pain exerted by the head is made visible, almost tangible, through the clasping of the patients' fingers across her skull. Thus, participants themselves produce a sense of object agency in and through action and interaction, entailing action in objects in the course of their presentation of those objects.

One aspect of the delight of these demonstrations is the ways in which they are designed with regard to the circumstances at hand and particularly the emerging co-participation of the recipients. To address their design in any detail is beyond the scope of this book but it is perhaps worthwhile mentioning one brief point. In the first place it can be noted how a variety of bodily animations are organised with regard to the orientation and appreciation of the recipient. Some are nicely and obviously played within the natural focal area of the recipient's orientation. Others, if only by virtue of the location of the object or symptom, demand the speaker to reshape the visual orientation of the other to enable the gesture to establish its viewer and sequential significance (see Heath, forthcoming). Many of these demonstrations are not simply designed to provide an embodied portrayal of an envisioned-design-in-action or symptoms of suffering, but rather are simultaneously shaped to establish particular forms of co-orientation and participation. Note, for example, the recycling of the crab mime in Fragment 3.2 until the tutor begins to display appreciation of the action (see also Heath, 1986; Heath, 1989).

The materials discussed in this chapter raise a further issue of some sociological relevance and certainly a theme that arises in ethnomethodology and particularly the lectures of Harvey Sacks. In his analysis of stories in conversation, Sacks discusses the distinction between *describing* and *witnessing* events, and then explores various entitlements and implications of this distinction (Sacks, 1992). In the materials at hand we can see how the participants, in the course of describing an object or their suffering, attempt to reconfigure the ways in which the co-participant(s) gain a sense of the object in question. Rather than simply hearing a description, the co-participants are provided with the opportunity to witness, see for themselves, just the ways in which the object might be used or the illness experienced. Thus, the local audience are confronted with the briefcase in use or the body inflicting pain and suffering. The speakers, students or patients, design their characterisation to enable others to see for themselves, what they see and experience; to experience first-hand the possibilities and experiences associated with the phenomena in question.

Acknowledgements

We appreciate the support and input of Jason Cleverly and our thanks are due to all the participants for allowing us to film them and publish our research. An earlier version of the chapter was presented at the Cardiff Roundtable on Discourses of the Body and we are very grateful to all the participants for their valuable comments on the work. The written version of the text has received valuable comment from Justine Coupland and Richard Gwyn, Neil Jenkings, Barry Brown and Dirk vom Lehn and useful contributions have been provided by various members of the WIT research group. This research has been supported by the ESRC (Award No. R000237136) and the EU SHAPE project (Award No. 26069).

Notes

1. All names have been changed to preserve anonymity.
2. Although full details are provided by Jefferson, it may be worth very briefly describing the key symbols for the purposes at hand. Talk is presented turn by turn, pauses and silences are captured in tenths of a second and included in brackets; '(.)' indicates a mini-pause, less than two-tenths of a second; underlinings show that a word or part of a word is emphasised; colons indicate that the prior sound is elongated; square brackets before turns indicate overlapping talk, '*hhh' preceded by an asterisk indicate an in breath, without an asterisk, outbreath. All transcripts have been simplified where reasonable to assist clarity.

References

Büscher, M. (2001) *Ideas in the Making: Talk, Vision, Objects and Embodied Action in Multi-media Art and Landscape Architecture.* Ph.D thesis.

Büscher, M. and Shapiro, D. (2000) *Vision at Work.* London: Queen Mary & Westfield.

Emerson, J. (1970) 'Behaviour in Private Places: Sustaining Definitions of Reality in Gynecological Examinations', in H.P. Dreitzel (ed.) *Recent Sociology.* New York: Macmillan.

Goodwin, C. (1981) *Conversational Organisation: Interaction between Speakers and Hearers.* London: Academic Press.

Goodwin, C. in press 'Pointing as a Situated Practice'. In S. Kita (ed.) *Pointing: Where Language, Culture and Cognition Meet.* Hillsdale, NJ: Lawrence Erlbaum Associates.

Goodwin, C. (1994) 'Professional Vision' *American Anthropologist* 96(3): 606–33.

Goodwin, C. (1995) 'Seeing in Depth' *Social Studies of Science* 25(2, May): 237–74.

Goodwin, C. and Goodwin, M.H. (1992) *Professional Vision.* Plenary Lecture Presented at the International Conference on Discourse and the Professions, Uppsala, Sweden, August 28, 1992.

Greatbatch, D., Luff, P., Heath, C.C. and Campion, P. (1993) 'Interpersonal Communication and Human–Computer Interaction: an Examination of the Use of Computers in Medical Consultations'. *Interacting with Computers* 5(2): 193–216.

Heath, C.C. (1986) *Body Movement and Speech in Medical Interaction.* Cambridge: Cambridge University Press.

Heath, C.C. (forthcoming) 'Demonstrative Suffering: The Gestural (Re)embodiment of Symptoms' *Journal of Communication.*

Heath, C.C. (1989) 'Pain Talk: the Expression of Suffering in the Medical Consultation' *Social Psychology Quarterly* 52(2): 113–25.

Heath, C.C. (1992) The Delivery and Reception of Diagnosis in the General Practice Consultation', in Talk at Work: Interaction in Institutional Settings, Drew, P. and Heirtage, J. (eds) Cambridge University Press, 235–67.

Heath, C.C. and Hindmarsh, J. (2002) 'Analysing Interaction: Video, ethnography and situated conduct', in T. May (ed.) *Qualitative Research: An International Guide to Practice.* London: Sage, 99–121.

Heath, C.C. and Hindmarsh, J. (2000) 'Configuring Action in Objects: From Mutual Space to Media Space', *Mind, Culture and Activity* 7(1/2): 81–104.

Heath, C.C. and Luff, P.K. (2000) *Technology in Action.* Cambridge: Cambridge University Press.

Heritage, J.C. (1984) *Garfinkel and Ethnomethodology.* Cambridge: Polity Press.

Hindmarsh, J. and Heath, C. (2000) 'Embodied Reference: A Study of Deixis in Workplace Interaction'. *Journal of Pragmatics* 32: 1855–78.

Hindmarsh, J. and Heath, C. (2000) 'Sharing the Tools of the Trade: The Interactional Constitution of Workplace Objects'. *Journal of Contemporary Ethnography* 29(5): 523–62.

Hirschauer, S. (1991) 'The Manufacture of Bodies in Surgery', *Social Studies of Science* 21: 279–319.

Jefferson, G. (1984) 'Transcript Notation', in J.M. Atkinson and J. Heritage (eds) *Structures of Social Action: Studies in Conversation Analysis*. Cambridge: Cambridge University Press, ix–xvi.

Kendon, A. (1982) 'The Organization of Behavior in Face-to-Face Interaction: Observations on the Development of a Methodology', in K. Scherer and P. Ekman (eds) *Handbook of Methods in Nonverbal Behavior Research*. Cambridge: Cambridge University Press.

Kendon, A. (2000) 'Language and Gesture: Unity of Duality?' in D. McNeil (ed.) *Language and Gesture*. Cambridge: Cambridge University Press.

Latour, B. (1992) 'Where are the Missing Masses? The Sociology of a Few Mundane Artifacts', in W.E. Bijker and J. Law (eds) *Shaping Technology/Building Society: Studies in Sociotechnical Change*. Cambridge, MA: MIT Press.

LeBaron, C. and Streeck, J. (2000) 'Gestures, Knowledge, and the World', in D. McNeil (ed.) *Language and Gesture*. Cambridge: Cambridge University Press.

Marx, K. (1977) *Economic and Philosophic Manuscripts of 1844*. Moscow: Progress Publishers.

Mead, G.H. (1934) *Mind, Self and Society*. Chicago: University of Chicago Press.

Paterson, M. *Haptic Spaces*. PhD thesis in preparation.

Sacks, H. (1992) *Lectures in Conversation: Volumes I and II*. Oxford: Blackwell.

Streeck, J. (1996) 'How To Do Things With Things: Objets Trouvés and Symbolization'. *Human Studies* 19(4): 365–84.

Wieder, D.L. (1974) 'Telling the Code', in R. Turner (ed.) *Ethnomethodology*. Harmondsworth: Penguin.

Wootton, A.J. (1994) 'Object Transfer, Intersubjectivity and Third Person Repair: Early Developmental Observations of One Child'. *Journal of Child Language* 21: 543–64.

4
Flirting
Alan Radley

Introduction

This chapter explores the discursive and non-discursive potential of the body through a consideration of flirtation. I choose to raise this topic because it questions treating the body as primarily the object of discourse. I also question the notion that the body might somehow lie outside discourse altogether, meaning that it is not subject to how people think and talk about social life. Instead, this chapter acknowledges that flirtation is possible only because people employ discourse to frame their actions. However, more important still, it argues that flirting is done only by people who are embodied (who *are*, not just *have* bodies), and that this crucially involves the use of symbolic gesture. This means that any consideration of this topic must take due account of how people flirt, not just what they say about, or even during, flirting. The act of flirting must necessarily involve knowledge practices, and with that the idea of a discourse of sexuality, so that the schemes involved here can well be thought of as discursively ordered. In that case, why choose flirting rather than some other social activity? The simple answer is that flirting involves the body in ways that many other activities do not. Flirting directly implicates the body at two levels, as it were, as being both the medium and the object of communication. The other's body conveys messages about his or her desirability, where that desirability is literally grounded in the potential of bodies to touch and to enfold. And yet, as we shall see below, flirting is premised upon neither the necessity nor even the likelihood that the two bodies in question will ever come into (sexual) contact. This means that while the 'physicality' of the body is crucial to flirtation, it does not enter into this scheme in a strictly 'physical' sense. Whatever is going on here is a matter of symbolic communication. Choosing this topic gives us an opportunity to rediscover 'the body' in a different frame to that where its physicality is taken as a given, as a 'take it or leave it' entity in relation to discourse.

In addition, there is the extended, metaphoric potential of the word 'flirtation'. We speak of people flirting with death, with their work, or with a simple pastime like cooking. This sense contrasts this way of doing (or not doing?) with the idea of commitment, of taking things seriously. There is, then, more than a passing resemblance between flirtation and play, implying the opposition between flirting and seriousness, or even power. So, to examine flirtation is perhaps to do more than analyse a specific bodily act. It might also question the assumption that we should direct our inquiries primarily or even exclusively to the way that people control, identify, or represent their world – in effect, in some way to fix it. As Adam Phillips has put it:

> To be committed to something – a person, an ideology, a vocabulary, a way of going about things – one has to be committed, perhaps unconsciously, to commitment itself. The question need not be: should we dispense with our capacity for commitment? But, what does commitment leave out of the picture that we might want?
>
> (1994: xviii)

There are a number of ways of addressing this question of what commitment might 'leave out of the picture'. One is to study acts of commitment (and its avoidance) in discourse, so as to reveal the ways that people rhetorically construct notions of flirtation, and use these as ways of proposing and legitimating various lines of argument. For example, Edwards (1995) has shown how, in conversation, a couple used the idea of flirtation to argue about whether the woman 'is a flirt'. This label is treated as a charge to be made and countered by the couple concerned in the course of establishing what is expected and proper in everyday socialising. This is a good example of the discursive approach, where an analysis of talk is used to unfold how people constitute what shall count as flirtation, and what this means in the context of accounting for the legitimacy of one's actions. From this perspective, it is mistaken to treat flirtation as a set of behaviours that are invoked at particular times to aid in gaining a partner. Discursive psychology moves to a position where language is conceived, not as a template for ordering an inchoate world, but in terms of 'talk and texts as part of social practices' (Potter, 1996).

This seems to me a perfectly proper position to take, as long as one emphasises the words 'as part of'. Clearly, it is possible to explore the way that people talk about such things as emotions, and the social situations in which they are deemed appropriate or even demanded (Harré and Gillet, 1994). However, it is unsatisfactory to be left either with the option of studying flirtation-talk or else with examining the cultural construction of flirtation as a wholly conventionalised activity – 'when' it means, 'to whom' it means, and 'why'. Either of these approaches is acceptable up to the point where we want to ask questions about the act as significant gesture. This perhaps should be rephrased to ask, what are the modes of representation employed in the act of flirtation and to what end is discourse employed during flirtation? By this I mean, how do flirtatious gestures signify as they are executed by embodied individuals, in the context of their meeting, as these acts might fleetingly appear? The reason for asking this question is, first, to re-examine the question of the relationship of the body to discourse, and second to stake a claim for flirtation as an exemplar of a way of being (of thinking, talking, acting) that current schemes of discourse analysis overlook.

Before beginning our discussion of flirtation, it is important to say something about the terms being used in this chapter, particularly concerning the body. To speak about 'the body' in relation to 'discourse' runs the risk of being seen to set up an opposition that sets relativist against realist. This situation occurs because this terminology sets apart language and embodied existence in a way that either allocates separate powers to these two aspects of human existence or else allocates all power to language. One way of dealing with this is to take apart the rhetoric on which realist arguments are based, so that questions of the body remain always questions of (linguistic) construction (Edwards, Ashmore and Potter, 1995). But there is a problem with this approach, for it appears to deny the reality of the body. In order to counter this implication, Potter (1996) has argued that the intention is not to deny the existence of bodies, but to decouple the implied equivalence between relativism and lack of political commitment. In a recent further attempt at clarification, Edley (2001) points out that talking about such things as emotions is constitutive of how we understand ourselves as emotional beings. This means that flirting and the feelings associated with it would be, 'in the *ontological* sense of construction', a 'consequence of the terms we apply to ourselves' (*ibid*.: 438).

Now, there can be no doubt that flirting involves cultural schemes (discourses) for the making of social and sexual contacts, and that these have consequences. Even saying this moves the notion of discourse on from language to the ordered practices wherein issues of power and resistance are worked through in relationships. However, this still leaves open the question as to how flirtation, with its characteristic non-commitment, is fabricated in the course of action. It also leaves unexamined the place of the body in flirtation, in the sense of ascribing to its various potentialities some role in the making of meaning that this involves. To do this one has to break out of the idea that light can only be thrown on discourse by looking at where discourse is focally illuminated (namely on language).

I want to criticise the assumption that, because anything done or felt must be spoken to be analysed, these things must not only be knowable within discourse, but *as discourse*. This forces the choice either to remove matters of the body to that plane, or to leave them in the sphere of (unknowable) things. Like 'questions of commitment', I shall argue that this choice is not the issue we ought to consider, and if we want to know about embodiment, it is not at all the best one to pose. This is because embodiment – as the condition for human action – is not to be confused with 'the body' taken as a physical entity. To confuse the two terms – or rather to assimilate embodiment to physicality – is to bracket out, from the beginning, the possibility that there are ways of symbolising other than using discourse. By discourse I mean primarily, but not only, the use of language – effectively what might be spelled out in words. Exactly what I mean by things bracketed out in the course of discursive analyses is the main concern of what follows in this chapter.

To anticipate what is to come, my argument is that 'the body', primarily the *object* of the discourse perspective, must be abandoned as focus if we are to entertain ideas about embodiment and its signifying potential.

On flirtation

Flirtation employs both words and actions. Rather than being just an example of individual behaviour, it is more a description of a social activity. Or rather, to flirt is to invoke or to invite a change of social relationship, so that whatever flirting 'is' owes as much to what it makes possible as to what enables it to occur. This disclaimer is not meant to cloud a common experience, a widely practised capacity. We all know how to flirt even if we are not all experts at it. And we all know what it is to be flirted *with* even if we are not equally sensitive to the message being given out. As a result one might try to say what actions are involved in this activity. But to say this, in the sense of denoting what is done (for example flirting is when you touch someone's hand, or flutter your eyelids, or use a soft tone of voice, or propose a discreet meeting), actually misses the point of it all. We can attempt to describe flirting, but better to illustrate it. Imagine reading the following:

'Just hold the torch a moment', she said, 'while I look for the key.'
'How am I expected to do that?' he replied, 'with an armful of books?'
'Easy.' She pushed the torch gently towards his mouth so that he grasped it between his teeth. He stood with his head on one side, angling the beam, while she groped in her bag for the key. Once she had opened the door he staggered in, still clutching the books. Before switching on the light she took the torch from him, waiting for him to open his mouth, so that for a moment the beam played about the room, giving him a glimpse of her reaching for the switch on the wall. 'There, that wasn't so bad, was it?' she said, as he stood blinking at her over the pile of books he was still holding.

Try to analyse this little piece in terms of discrete behaviours and one is in for a hard time in terms of saying exactly what is flirtatious in it. Putting a torch in another person's mouth? Hardly. Speaking to someone in a slightly condescending manner? Possibly, but not really a sufficient condition. One answer might be that the piece only appears flirtatious in the context of this chapter, one that flags up this particular reading as salient. Hence, what is invited is a reading in terms of socially available schemes or discourses about gender relationships as described in novels. While this is inescapable, I would also say that any 'flirtatious' reading of the description lies in drawing the reader's attention away from the use of objects in the interplay between the two people concerned. Something here is expressive of the mood of the moment. But what, and how is the body involved in this?

To answer these points I want to turn to the work of the nineteenth-century German sociologist Georg Simmel (1984). He pointed out that the essence of flirtation lies precisely in a refusal of commitment, made possible by sustaining an antithesis of accommodation and denial. In what might be thought its banal form, the flirtatious gesture of the sidelong glance with the head half-turned accedes in its momentary acceptance of the other, while also hinting at aversion in its refusal to make face-to-face contact. This is not a static juxtaposition, but is constructed through a mutual interplay of the two possibilities. This means that refusal in flirtation is never absolute, but pregnant with the possibility of acceptance, while invitations are made *sotto voce*, or covertly, or by reference to a third party. This latter condition shows that flirtation is neither open invitation nor merely an attempt at seduction. Strictly speaking, to flirt is *not* to try to overcome, either by force or by seduction. Simmel (1984) described flirtation as involving 'an allusive dissent', in which there is evoked an ambiguous sense of the ability *and* the inability to acquire something. There is a displacement away from the sphere of real desires to a world of virtual powers, a kind of 'taking aside' in which suggestion and the suspension of decision play important roles.

Flirting, as with playing, invokes a sense of time and place that conjures an illusory fragment of experience torn from the broad fabric of everyday life. This is achieved where the action communicates the symbol of an idea rather than the symptom of desire. One crucial element in this is the way that things might be shown, or be partly revealed, or perhaps concealed. This way of showing/concealing is central to the nature of flirtation. It has the effect of making what is concealed both more noticeable and worthy of attention. It also has the effect of making it appear that the person 'acts from a remote distance' (Simmel, 1984: 134) so that the mode of reference, avoiding direct reference, is one of allusion. As well as by concealment, this operates through utilising extraneous objects – items of clothing, household items – which as the object of attention allow something important to take place. In what might be called a description of 'deep flirtation' (Geertz, 1972), Zola tells how Nana's suitors were captivated by being allowed to watch her at her toilette, by the very range of powders and rouge which she made use of in her preparations. Such objects provide the means whereby the flirt can give shape to his or her desire, being a focus that allows the realisation of a performance showing what attentions might be bestowed upon the admirer. In the course of this, there is a transformation in the meaning of these everyday physical objects, so that articles of clothing, possessions or even trinkets take on a special meaning for the parties concerned. And, of course, the telephone can be a special means for flirtation. Here, a prosthetic technology affords whispers and modulations of the voice that fashion a special presence for the words that are uttered. 'The body' extends beyond the physical bodies of the parties concerned, to eroticise and colonise the world that they re-make in the act of flirtation.

In its refusal of commitment, flirtation shares a number of features that are often associated with play, not least the fact that the pleasure obtained comes from the practice of flirtation itself. This underlines the point made earlier, that to flirt is not to seduce; it is not a means to an end, even though that end might eventually be forthcoming. This parallel with play is seen in the fact that flirtation is something that can be done well or badly, and that the suspense of 'having and not-having' which is key to its form is premised upon there being no resolution of this contradiction in the course of the action. Flirtation, like play, is fragile, open to the complicity of others who are invited to enter into it, and subject to being terminated by responses that, not recognising it for being what it is, confuse its symbols with signs relating to sexual provocation or denial. Flirtation is destroyed by the insistence on commitment, by the need to have a definitive 'yes' or a 'no' as answer. It can even be undermined by the open acknowledgement that it is taking place, where this reduces its allusive qualities to the literal (that is, the exchange is then seen as 'inappropriate'). Finally, as with play, flirtation achieves its form by virtue of taking up, or in some way altering the objects of the mundane world. How this is achieved will be dealt with at some length below. As Simmel put it, 'While it is true that flirtation also does no more than play with reality, yet it is still *reality* with which it plays' (1984: 145, emphasis in the original). What Simmel meant by 'reality' here is open to interpretation, but his point was that flirtation makes its appearance in the world, not over and above it. For the purposes of this chapter, what is important is that it is by virtue of our being embodied that flirtation makes its appearance at all. How is this possible and what might this mode of signification tell us about the relationship of embodiment to discourse?

Expression and denotation

In one of his earliest publications, dealing with symbols of class status, Goffman (1951) distinguished between what he termed their 'categorial' and 'expressive' significance. By categorial symbols, Goffman meant those signifiers concerned with denoting identity or membership. In the context of social class these might denote the individual as 'middle-class', effectively invoking a boundary condition to specify the person as a member of a particular group. In comparison, the 'expressive' mode of signification refers not to identity but to a more general kind of potential. Goffman's chosen example was duelling in past ages, which he claimed was largely redundant as a marker of social class (only being engaged in by the gentry) but was effective in portraying a particular style of life. This style of life – of a man prepared to face danger in defence of his self-respect – was important in its potential to inspire all of the man's actions, whatever they might be.

Later on, Goffman (1959) used this distinction in his seminal treatise on self-presentation, where the idea of 'giving-off' information was made a crucial complement to the way in which identities are not just asserted ('given', denoted). This was explained by showing that a person's 'self' must be claimed through effective performances, which are not reducible to natural expressions, but are forms of what he later termed 'social portraiture' (Goffman, 1976). In making this point, Goffman tried to explain how, for example, men and women either might comply with or depart from the accepted social schedules defining masculinity and femininity to portray their gender identity. From this position, the question of flirtation might be posed in terms of socially defined schedules of courtship appropriate to the sexes. And yet to do so hardly takes us further than saying that flirtation is a possible way of being in relation to a desired other, either of the opposite or of the same sex. In effect, to make the question of portrayal into a matter of whether one endorses or denies social schedules of action loses the potential of the idea of expression that Goffman originally drew out (see Radley, 1996, for a more extended consideration of this point).

Goodman (1968) has, I think, come closest to saying precisely what is going on in performances that are deemed expressive. For him the essential issue is that denotation symbolises by pointing to something as a member of a class, so that the predicate describes by classifying, by inscribing. This can involve naming something, or else pointing to something (with one's foot perhaps) and sometimes doing both at the same time. Clearly, denotation is a mode of signification that is common to both speech and action. Goodman contrasts denotation with a different mode of signification, that of exemplification. Exemplification is a form of reference in which, say, a picture or a person stands as a sample of that to which it (s/he) refers. This involves, at one time, both having properties and referring to them. Hence, a sketch, like a poem, can be contrasted to a script or a musical score in that 'it does not so much define a work ... but rather *is* one' (Goodman, 1968: 193, emphasis in the original).

Given the above, what are normally referred to as 'expressions' (cries) of pain, anger or sexual pleasure are not expressions as I am using the term here. These are, instead, the literal symptoms of different states of physical being. Instead, what embodied people express are ideas, not movements. To flirt is to exemplify a situation, a way of being, by showing forth those properties deemed essential to it. It is not, therefore, merely to act in a way that is constituted (as a schedule) by those properties, for this would merely be to have and to show them. Instead, flirting is defined as an expressive act through being exemplary of the properties it shows forth, but which are not intrinsic to those movements. That is why no study of (just) the prescribed movements of flirting could ever reach an understanding of what makes this a humanly significant and psychologically interesting activity. (The parallel here is, of course, an attempt to understand art only through a specification of the distribution of the paint or other medium.)

However, this is not to say that a person cannot exemplify as well as be denoted – so that a man who aligns himself with the culturally understood scheme of 'manliness', and so acts that way, also exemplifies that condition. But the mere alignment with a scheme is insufficient to be expressive, for this is only to display those features of manliness that properly belong to the accepted cultural definition. In saying this I don't mean to imply that 'features of manliness' are physical (what some would call 'natural') aspects of gender role. These features of gender role behaviour are cultural patternings too, as Mauss (1972) taught us long ago. The point is that aligning ourselves with them – endorsing them if you will – in the way we walk, gesture and use our bodies is to be an example of a man (or woman) walking but is not expressive of anything else. It is not that walking cannot be expressive but that it has to be made to be so. But I make these distinctions for the purpose of clarifying terms: they are not to be found separately in everyday life. Goffman's point about categorial and expressive symbols was that these are found in the *same* displays of action, not separated out into isolated pieces of behaviour.

The relevance of the above commentary is that expressive meanings are not isolated from alignments, from denotation. Indeed, displays are often the subject of discourse, so that we may talk about flirtation, and we may even categorise people into better and worse flirts if we wish. By refusing to acknowledge flirting or play we can deny them. But neither naming nor shaming expressive acts removes them from the plane of embodiment, still less explains them.

This distinction between denotation and exemplification, and the consequent involvement of portrayal or display in expression, is potentially of great value for understanding flirtation. It takes us beyond notions that this is an act solely derivative of sexual desire; that it is intended primarily to identify oneself with a particular social group; or even, as we shall see below, that it is a form of social interaction designed to control or coerce the other. It also dismisses, at a stroke, the notion that in some way these two forms of symbolising are each, in their turn, identifiable with discourse and with the physical body. In doing this it also challenges the assumption that, in the analysis of flirtation, discourse and body must be treated as separate entities.

Flirtation as performance

Flirting, like other expressive acts, symbolises through portrayal. To flirt is to exemplify, but to exemplify what? We have said that flirtation is misunderstood if reduced to being the prelude to seduction, even though that might, in some circumstances, be the eventual conclusion. The idea that flirting involves both showing and hiding, invitation and refusal, must necessarily be achieved in the course of gesture being negated as a symptom of desire. In this it shares something important with playfulness, which activity has at its core the refusal of commitment. This refusal extends to a negation of the situation as 'serious', as something that can be framed definitively, that names it as a this or a that situation. This is not a matter of definition, merely, but one of exemplifying through a transformation of what is at hand. To be exemplary, flirting (like playing) involves a sustained performance that transforms the situation by engaging it. We do not flirt through speech and action – but *with* words and *with* our bodies. In the case of the second, this relies upon making differences not only in our gestures but also in the material world that we inhabit.

Play and flirtation involve a double-consciousness of the transposition of the mundane by the imaginary, and of the fabrication of the imaginary on the basis of the mundane. This double involvement is the experiential parallel to Goodman's (1968) argument that expressive symbolism runs in two directions simultaneously – from the predicate to the object and from the object to the predicate. So, for example, a picture denotes something (a grey sea) and yet in being seen to exemplify the sea's character might itself be apprehended (metaphorically) as 'a disturbing picture'. It is only secondarily (though literally) a 'grey picture'. So, too, with flirtation. It is by exemplification – through performative display – that the flirt's actions are experienced as expressive of the relationship in which they are fabricated.

The kinds of gesture normally understood to be involved (e.g., the sidelong glance) are indicative of the way in which the body is used in flirting. And the reference to dress and other objects in the course of flirtation reinforces the idea that this activity does not just take place 'in context', nor even defines context, but actually fabricates it. To flirt is to define a world of possibility (expressive potential) through engaging another in a jointly constructed time and space. In this it is not unlike ritual where, as Geertz (1972) so eloquently put it concerning the Balinese cockfight, the purpose of the physical trappings is neither to assuage nor to heighten passions, but to display them. Flirtation, like ritual, *is a way of seeing the world differently*, of entertaining it as if it were or could be different.

Therefore, as with metaphor, flirtation separates the virtual from the mundane. But as with metaphor, it does this only to join them in creating a world of possibility, in which the play of imagination is shown in the fragments of movement or of glances. It is therefore illustrative of a way of symbolising. It is neither more (nor less) an act peculiar to the physical body than it is a cultural scheme for inviting intimacy. Instead, this discussion shows that the distinction made between denotation and expression provides a more powerful way of analysing issues to do with 'discourse and the body' than is provided by taking the separation of these two terms at face value. Clearly, the body can denote (by pointing) and language can express (through poesis), as well as the other way round. Also, we can call a person a flirt, or we can say to a person 'I am flirting with you'. But neither of these (denotative) statements satisfies the criterion (of expressive form) for it being an act of flirting that is understood as such.

The limitation of seeing flirting as primarily denotation extends to any explanation that would see it as just another form of metacommunication. Bateson made this kind of analysis with respect to play, where he observed that monkeys initiate play by nipping each other, just as humans signal lightheartedness by giving someone a slap on the back. The question is, how is the nip to be read? For Bateson, it read, 'this nip which denotes a bite does not denote what a bite would normally denote' (1987: 180). He saw the nip as a metacommunication that signalled a change in the mode of communication – to be read as 'this is play'. However, this leaves as mysterious the difference in denotation, which as a problem arises within the context of an adult human observer looking at simians or children. The essential point is not that the nip *denotes* a bite differently, but that it is *part of a display* that exemplifies a mode of being (playfulness) that can be referred back as a descriptor of the performance. In saying 'this is play', the nip comes to denote (metacommunicate, frame) the sphere of play but first says, presentationally, self-referentially, 'THIS is play'. And in the same way, I contend, does flirting communicate the message, 'Shall we flirt?' by virtue of saying, 'THIS is flirting'.

The elusory nature of flirtation

In this section I want to deal with two important features of flirtation as an expressive act. One concerns the locus of meaning of the acts performed, particularly in relation to whether expression is a function of 'the body'. The other concerns the elusory nature of this way of signifying. These two ideas are connected, and together have important implications for the way that we consider the issue of 'discourse and the body'.

The first point I will take up is that flirtation, being dramatically portrayed, fabricates the time and space in which it occurs. This is another way of saying that flirting (like playing) not only takes time – which it does – but *makes time*, in that it has virtual qualities seemingly deriving from the imaginary world that is conjured. We should avoid the idea that this is some ethereal issue, when the point is that, as embodied creatures, we impinge upon the material world. What is a caress but a touch extended? This is what it is (and what it is not) – by virtue of that resistance and reception characterising the body's sensory layer. Following Merleau-Ponty's (1962) proposals about the body, we can say that it is by virtue of our double existence – in the virtual and the mundane together – that the imaginary is found in the mundane, now transformed. Like the space–time of play (Winnicot, 1971), flirtation may be fragile and easily disrupted. The present it creates is experienced, in spatio-temporal terms, as being a series of *particular engagements*, which nevertheless symbolise an extensive possibility or way of being. This extensive possibility embraces Goffman's (1951) notion of a style of life, a term used to cover expression as a mode signifying what one might term a virtual world. For the flirt – and for the other who is flirted with – this world of delights and sensibilities is at once fragile and pregnant with possibility. And yet it is also a 'here and now', being portrayed in the course of a performance whose allusion to this wider sphere lends significance to the specifics of what is said and done. The act of flirtation is therefore expressive in the sense that, like a picture, it alludes to an imaginary world that at the same time lends significance and coherence to the specifics that constitute its portrayal. Therefore, while flirtation is irreducible to movement (and hence to 'the body' considered as a physical entity), it makes its appearance by virtue of modulations of the world that we inhabit as embodied individuals. This is not least because flirtation 'plays with' desire, and with the possibilities that can only be entertained by individuals with sensuous bodies.

The second point to be made follows from the idea that expressive acts signify by allusion, involving a 'taking aside' of the mundane, be this the 'real world' or the body's 'real desires'. In relation to flirting, this means that it is those features of talk and action that lend themselves to allusion and ambiguity that are most useful in its achievement. This is because it would not be better done (or be better shown) if one could point directly at its meanings, or if one could render the ambiguous wholly visible. As Simmel so perceptively pointed out, flirtation 'lends a positive concreteness to not-having, making it tangible for the first time by means of the playful, suggestive illusion of having' (1984: 150). Not only is it a mistake to attempt to describe flirtation in terms of denotation alone, but it is equally mistaken to attempt to denote that which is better recognised as being allusive. To do so is to treat expressive acts as if they hid 'something' that could better be rendered in words. This potential error is not limited to treatments of flirtation, but to all theories that presume an entity called 'the body' that awaits disclosure. Merleau-Ponty made this clear in considering 'literature, music and the passions', which, he said, are unlike the ideas of science because 'they cannot be detached from the sensible appearances and be erected into a second positivity' (1968: 149). Instead, this form of expression, he argues, is 'their proper mode of existence'. To flirt and to be flirted with depend upon this elusory feature of action, which has to be acknowledged if we are not to fall into the trap of thinking that flirting is located *either* in physical movement *or* in the social world.

Instead, flirtation belongs to what Langer (1957) called 'virtual gestures', to distinguish them from gestures relating to cries of pain or pleasure. The concept of gesture is important in pointing up once more the difference between portrayal and naming as ways of signifying. Flirtatious gestures are culturally shaped, but their primary function is not to point to things outside the sphere that they create. Instead, they are effective insofar as they display their world all the better. (For a parallel argument in relation to religious painting, see Latour, 1998). This means that to enjoy flirting is not to see what these gestures point towards, but to appreciate in their presentational form a meaning that depends upon the embodied engagement of the Other. It is for this reason that apparent elusiveness is not just a feature of the flirt's performance. Instead, it is contributed to by our (the Other's) co-participation in the act, as we take up the invitation to 'make the world' in this way. This 'making as' is more than a perceptuo-motor act. As Merleau-Ponty says, 'The whole difficulty is to conceive this act clearly without confusing it with a cognitive operation' (1962: 185). I would add to this that difficulty remains if one tries to conceive of it as simply a denotative act, in terms of naming or interpreting gesture by discursive means. It is only comprehensible once one conceives of the Other as endorsing or accepting the flirt's invitation to 'take aside' the realities of desire. In a sense, flirtation only properly appears once the Other recognises the invitation in the actor's gesture. Whether or not we wish to call this a 'taking over' of expressive gesture is less important than the recognition that to understand flirtation is not, first, to name it but to endorse it. Of course, once experienced, flirtation *can* be named, as in the case of seeing someone flirt with a third party. But this is to denote 'the act of flirting', not to be co-complicit with it. Flirting is an act that cannot be analysed in full, or in Merleau-Ponty's terms, be erected into a second positivity. However, one should not confuse this acknowledgement of the *elusory* potential of embodiment (the act that cannot be analysed in full) with the *elusiveness* of the body that escapes discourse (Radley, 1995). Flirting uses both speech and practical schemes of sexual relationships ('non-verbal behaviours'), so that it employs discourse to fashion the 'imaginary world' in which its participants exist, precariously, fugitively, for perhaps a very short time. But to say only that this makes it 'discursive' or that there is a 'discourse of flirtation' is to say virtually nothing at all.

Discourse and the body: some implications

This analysis shows a quite different relationship of 'discourse to body' from that presumed by the view that discourse somehow 'constructs' the body. It is undoubtedly true that gestures are culturally formed, so that flirtation, as one example of the use of gesture, is itself a cultural way of acting. And this means that to understand flirtation, to know what is or might be intended by another, is only possible because we share certain cultural understandings about action and its boundaries. Treated as a text, these gestures can be explained by means of discourses of sexuality and gender relations. We might say that such discourses inhabit the text, or that by rendering what is done into spoken or written form makes the concept of discourse appropriate if not central (Parker, 1990).

However, the proposition that the body – or gesture – is a text waiting to be explained in words presumes a particular relationship of interpretation of the problematic. It suggests that the body is knowable only by being spoken about. This is an unwarrantable limitation on the possibility that there might be other ways of knowing. They signify by showing forth, not by denotation aimed at naming and the articulation of signs. They also depend upon *not specifying* as a key aspect of communicating a way of being in the world. This does not mean 'not saying', because speech is one medium through which we can give expressive form to ideas of the possible. And flirtation is, as I have argued elsewhere (Radley, 1996), one example of the use of gesture in the fabrication of 'social worlds', considered as possible ways of being.

So, flirtation is not only about 'the body', any more than poetry is only about 'speech'. Neither of these concerns the outpouring of 'inner feelings', but instead symbolises its aim by portrayals that depend, in their immediacy, upon the use of recognisable cultural forms to fabricate their meaning (mainly gestures in one case, primarily language in the other). 'Good' poetry and flirtation 'done well' achieve their aims through establishing and sustaining a kind of ascetic distance, so that in each case we may speak of an art of good practice. To some extent we may understand each of these by analysing the detail of the gestures or the structure of the writing. This is possible because both forms of expression are sustained by virtue of being portrayed 'in' the words or gestures concerned, though in each case the significant meaning concerned cannot actually be located in either medium. To attempt to do so falls back into a confusion of expression with denotation that tries to reduce all that is known to what can be named. One cannot flirt without gesture in the same sense that one cannot write poetry without words, nor can one paint a picture without applying paint to canvas.

This way of thinking takes us beyond the notion that there is an entity called 'the body' that somehow has to be reconciled with discourse. Of course, it is perfectly possible to propose this separation of 'body' and 'discourse', but this must be seen for the assumptive act that it is. The posing of 'the body' as an entity separate from discourse is itself discursively produced. This is not a facile point but a rhetorical one, and is indicative of the primacy regularly given to denotative symbolisation in talk about the body. It has the effect of leading the argument back to the debate about realism versus construction, which argument either leaves the body outside discourse as an unknowable entity, or else includes in its vital powers only those things that can be spoken, that can be named. Both of these outcomes are unhelpful when we come to look at something like flirtation. For, on the one hand, we are left either with the idea that our embodied actions are wholly mysterious or, on the other, that they are nothing if they are not specifiable.

Even a brief study of flirtation shows this to be an untenable position. What is worthy of study is what is significant, and what is significant in flirtation is not just what is denoted but what is expressed. Expression involves a making of appearances that is aimed at not-specifying, that makes denotation (naming) necessary but insufficient. This, in turn, makes it possible for embodied acts (including talk) to become a symbolic veil, the occlusionary character of which *is* its meaning. If one attempts to undo this, to privilege one particular medium of communication (talk) over another (the body), then important ways of how we signify as embodied persons are rendered elusive (see also Hindmarsh and Heath, this volume). Then one has to return again and again to 'the body' to try to subjugate that which escapes specification. But, of course, it can never be wholly subjugated because 'the body' – with all its symbolic entrails – is the co-construction of the primacy of discourse as word: it is the 'Other', expelled ab-originally from the discourse perspective, forever agitating to be allowed back in.

I will try to finish on a more positive note. What I have argued is that flirtation involves discourse (if for no other reason than that flirting is done by speaking people!), but also that it makes its appearance through non-discursive symbols. These symbols are subject to conventionalisation as are verbal concepts, so that flirtation, as done, is culturally relative. If this were not so then how could it be learned? What is more important about flirtation is that its meanings are not achieved by denotation (description) alone, but through expression, and it is this distinction that is important for understanding how flirting is possible. The possibility here for 'not-commitment' is enabled by a kind of depiction, portrayal, that uses non-discursive gesture to make significant symbols. This capacity for portrayal is central to our powers to evoke a sphere of conjecture, and to invite and mutually endorse a 'way of life' that is virtual in the sense that it refigures the 'ordinary', the mundane. To flirt is to sketch a picture of a possible world, and it is worthy of our attention not for its peculiar qualities, but because it is just one example of a generalised capacity for 'non-commitment' that is integral with our being embodied speakers.

References

Bateson, G. (1987) *Steps to an Ecology of Mind*. Northvale, NJ: Jason Aronson.

Edley, N. (2001) 'Unravelling social constructionism'. *Theory & Psychology* 11: 433–41.

Edwards, D. (1995) 'Two to Tango: Script Formulations, Dispositions, and Rhetorical Symmetry in Relationship Troubles Talk'. *Research in Language and Social Interaction* 28: 319–50.

Edwards, D., Ashmore, M. and Potter, J. (1995) 'Death and Furniture: Arguments Against Relativism'. *History of the Human Sciences* 8: 25–49.

Geertz, C. (1972) 'Deep Play: Notes on the Balinese Cockfight'. *Daedalus* 101: 1–37.

Goffman, E. (1951) 'Symbols of Class Status'. *British Journal of Sociology* 2: 294–304.

Goffman, E. (1959) *The Presentation of Self in Everyday Life*. New York: Doubleday.

Goffman, E. (1976) 'Gender Advertisements'. *Studies in the Anthropology of Visual Communication* 3.

Goodman, N. (1968) *Languages of Art: an Approach to a Theory of Symbols*. Indianapolis: Bobbs-Merrill.

Harré, R. and Gillet, G. (1994) *The Discursive Mind*. London: Sage.

Langer, S.K. (1957) *Philosophy in a New Key: a Study in the Symbolism of Reason, Rite and Art*. 3rd edn. Oxford: Oxford University Press.

Latour, B. (1998) 'How to be Iconophilic in Art, Science and Religion?' In C. Jones and P. Galison (eds) *Picturing Science Producing Art*. New York: Routledge, 418–40.

Mauss, M. (1972) 'Techniques of the Body'. *Economy and Society* 2: 70–88.

Merleau-Ponty, M. (1962) *Phenomenology of Perception* (trans. Colin Smith). London: Routledge & Kegan Paul.

Merleau-Ponty, M. (1968) *The Visible and the Invisible*. Evanston: Northwestern University Press.

Parker, I. (1990) 'Discourse: Definitions and Contradictions'. *Philosophical Psychology* 3: 189–204.

Phillips, A. (1994) *On Flirtation*. London: Faber & Faber.

Potter, J. (1996) *Representing Reality: Discourse, Rhetoric and Social Construction*. London: Sage.

Radley, A. (1995) 'The Elusory Body and Social Constructionist Theory'. *Body & Society* 1(2): 3–23.

Radley, A. (1996) 'Displays and Fragments: Embodiment and the Configuration of Social Worlds'. *Theory & Psychology* 6: 559–76.

Simmel, G. (1984) *Georg Simmel: On Women, Sexuality and Love*. New Haven: Yale University Press.

Winnicot, D.W. (1971) *Playing and Reality*. London: Tavistock.

Part 2
Ideological Representations of the Body

5
Ageing Bodies: Aged by Culture

Mike Hepworth

Introduction

This chapter, divided into two parts, discusses the problem of the ageing body in an increasingly age-conscious society. The first part introduces the constructionist critique of the biomedical model of human ageing and the second part is an examination of Margaret Morganroth Gullette's radical critique of the 'decline narrative' in Western culture. For Gullette, the fact that the body changes biologically over time does not explain why ageing into old age should be widely perceived as a condition of psychological and social decline. In her view, biological change and decline are not synonymous: decline is a cultural construct epitomising the prevailing ageism of contemporary Western culture where the discursive consequences include the social marginalisation of older people and subjective experiences of insecurity and self-doubt in later life.

The biomedical model and the constructionist critique

In Western culture the master narrative of human ageing is biomedical and the biomedical model of ageing is essentially a reductionist model of decline. Sherwin B. Nuland (1997), for example, who teaches surgery and the history of medicine at Yale, argues for the cyclical evolutionary principle within each species of life; a continuous biologically determined process of continual regeneration and renewal. In the biomedical model, ageing is closely associated with decline (indeed, synonymous with it) because the cause of the physical debilitation associated with ageing into old age is perceived to be 'a general running down of normal structure and function' (*ibid.*: 72); a process of natural descent from a biological peak or zenith to dissolution and preparation for new growth.

Arguments for the essentially 'natural' or biomedical association of ageing with inevitable decline are widely contested by sociologists of ageing and of the body. But in proposing an alternative conceptualisation of decline it is important to stress that sociologists do not deny that ageing is a process of biological change; rather they wish to draw attention to the social and personal implications of the ways in which the meanings of biological change as 'decline' are culturally constructed and interpreted through discourse. In, for example, his Foucauldian analysis of the construction of knowledge of old age in the disciplines of geriatric medicine and gerontology, Stephen Katz (1996) has argued that the distinctive biomedical association of the ageing process with decline did not emerge entirely from the objective scientific scrutiny of the body in the mid-nineteenth century. The historical reality is that the ageing body was created as a biomedical discourse in the 'transformation from pre-modern to modern perceptions of the aged body' based upon medical reinterpretations of disease in terms of 'a new series of symptoms that constituted the aged body as a symbol of separation from other age groups' (*ibid.*: 40). During the nineteenth century the modern aged body was separated out from the body of youth and other stages of life as a degenerative or dying body:

> Whereas previous treatments for disease took little notice of age, modern treatments would depend upon it. The problem was less the health, vitality, or prolongevity of an elderly person than the progressively degenerative diseases that defined their state of ageing.
>
> (Katz: 41)

Fixation of the professional gaze upon the ageing body excluded visions of ageing as a complex 'polysemic' moral process involving interaction between 'the body and surfaces external to it' (*ibid.*: 40), concentrating attention on the embodied limits of physical existence. The ageing, dying body became the ultimate signifier of the 'limits of existence' moulding 'the aged person into a singular and finite subject' (*ibid.*: 42). The result was that the diverse human experience of ageing was gradually reduced to a single biomedical model of decline as defined by the unifying, disciplinary scrutiny of an expanding band of medical experts.

From the perspective of Foucauldian analysis, the emerging dominance of the biomedical model of ageing as decline is a discursive product of modernity – a model of the limitations imposed by what is currently understood to be the 'natural' human body. And it is at this point that sophisticated attempts in biomedicine to distinguish the degenerative consequences of diseases in later life from the 'normal' processes of ageing become apparent: the point at which efforts are made to conceptualise decline as a disease process and not an integral characteristic of the process of growing older as such. As Gubrium (1986) has argued in his classic study of the ways in which the diagnosis and understanding of Alzheimer's disease is descriptively organised through the use of language into a 'public culture' (*ibid.*: 111), considerable effort has been made in this field to separate processes of normal ageing from those associated with disease. In his view, the consciousness of growing older in a society that fears the association of ageing with decline generates considerable anxiety. The result is an intensification of effort to locate the causes of decline in pathology or disease and not in the 'normal' biological processes of ageing. If the problem of the ageing body can be traced to pathology, for example an empirically identifiable condition such as Alzheimer's Disease, then advances in biomedical knowledge of the body will ultimately provide a solution. As Gubrium puts it, biomedical definitions of the problem of the ageing body foster an 'adversarial attitude' or form of 'martial useage', which in turn encourages the belief that ageing should not, in the normal course of life, be a decremental bodily process endangering the unity of the body and the self. In the model of 'normal' disease-free ageing, the body and self are preserved in a state of harmonious unity. It is disease that threatens to separate the self from the body and the threat of this pathological separation is reflected in a 'public culture' of Alzheimer's Disease which includes images of the disease as the 'thief' of the self (*ibid.*: 43).

In this study of the social construction of 'public culture' of Alzheimer's Disease Gubrium argues this form of senile dementia 'conceptually stands in an uneasy relationship with normal ageing' because it is 'not yet clear whether the organic and behavioural markers of senility are features of a disease or of ageing' (*ibid.*: xi). The biomedical evidence that is used to establish boundaries between normal ageing and the effects of pathology (Alzheimer's Disease) is highly ambiguous. Yet, at the same time, the high level of anxiety over ageing provokes a frantic search for certainty and in a society that puts a high value on medical science it is 'natural' that we should turn to doctors for definitive descriptive categorisations of the distinctions between ageing and pathology. But the problem is that ageing is unlike disease in one significant respect: ageing is at once a universal, 'diverse', and yet 'vague' human condition:

> If the characteristics called ageing exist everywhere among older folk, it exists nowhere in particular; it is no thing. The categorical category called Alzheimer's disease, however, is described as existing only among certain elders and, thereby exists somewhere particularly; it is a distinctive thing.
>
> (Gubrium, 1986:49)

Gubrium sets out to expose key epistemological difficulties surrounding attempts to conceptualise the ageing as distinct from the diseased body in later life. The normally ageing body resists categorisation except in terms of the pathology made visible in the form of senile dementia, confusion and empirically observable difficulties with comprehension, self-expression, gesture, mobility and comportment.

The problem of defining ageing and old age can, as Bytheway (1985) has shown, be expressed in terms of the question 'How does old age exist at all?' What does the intending student of old age actually study and what are his/her sources of data? Any researcher into the origins and nature of old age is faced, Bytheway argues, with two difficulties. First, the problem of finding people who can speak informatively about old age and, secondly, of giving this material a perspective and coherence by relating it to the beliefs, theories and evidence that have already been published. In both cases the student is working with *words*. He/she is discovering the ways in which other people use such words as 'ageing', 'age' and 'old age' in everyday conversation and in professional and lay publications. According to this interpretation, the ageing body remains elusive and unsubstantiated:

> Without much difficulty, the student will find people who really admit to being old and who offer observations upon that condition. These will be valuable in that, if nothing else, students can learn something about how people use such terms as 'age' and 'old age' in everyday conversation. Before long, however, they will learn that few old people provide any explicit and direct information about what it is to be old. Few people are able to dissociate the role of being something from the role of observing themselves being that thing. As a consequence an old person's comments about being old are their comments about being what they are. Often their observations are relative: they compare how they are with how they were

yesterday, or last week or last year, or with how their spouses are or their neighbours, or with how they expected to be, or with how they might have been.

(Bytheway, 1985: 1–2)

But, persuasive though Bytheway's analysis may be, the older person is not always working with words *alone*. He or she is at some point using words to reflect on an embodied dilemma. When it comes to ageing, the intractable problem is that the body, as Nuland (1997) graphically shows, just won't go away. It is both elusory and substantial though not necessarily at one and the same time. Kathleen Woodward, (1991 and see her chapter in this volume), a cultural critic for whom words are equally important, has analysed the dilemma of the ageing body. If we live long enough there comes a time when we really are 'in' old age and there's no escape and biological embodiment claims us at the last. In Woodward's reading there comes a point when the constructive and reconstructive potential of words ultimately fails. She writes:

Ageing and old age are intimately related to biological phenomena. With the experience of the body being so central to the construction and experience of old age, I cannot agree with Bernice Neugarten that old age is an 'empty variable,' although I think her polemical assertion has done much to dispel stereotypes from the field of gerontology ... At best we may speak in the West of the compensations that may accompany the ordeals of old age, as did Bernard Berenson, for example, in his diaries, published under the title *Sunset and Twilight* ... But his experience also includes what he considers to be gifts of insight and gifts from others in old age. A certain kind of psychological work is implied.

(1991: 19)

As the last sentence in this quotation indicates, Woodward's reflection on the biological body as the bottom line in the ageing process does allow some space for compensatory 'psychological work'. And this is close to Arthur Frank's (1996) spirited defence of the potential for the 'reconciliatory alchemy' of the ailing body in the written word. Working primarily from assumptions derived from his personal experience of heart attack and testicular cancer, Frank proposes what he describes as 'a three-part relation between society, the body and the self' (1996: 53) in which the biological body, society and the self are reflexively interrelated. This relationship is so close that the three elements cannot ultimately be disentangled.

Simon Williams (1996), in his work on illness and the body, has described this complex reflexive interplay between the body, self and society as the 'vicissitudes of embodiment' where the word 'vicissitudes' indicates 'the alterations, fluctuations and mutability of our sense of embodiment' (*ibid.*: 24) He also takes the line that he is not questioning the 'fundamentally *embodied* nature of our human being' but rather that he is concerned with the 'phenomenological or experiential vicissitudes of embodiment across the chronic illness trajectory' and the implications of such bodily disruptions for 'our normal modes of bodily being' (*ibid.*: 24); see also Gwyn, this volume. He proposes a threefold processual model of embodiment, or body consciousness, where balances between the experience of the body and the self are neither fixed nor static but fluctuate over time.

In this model the first condition is embodiment: a condition of freedom from discomfort, illness or pain. This, as in Leder's (1990) concept of 'the absent body', is the experience of 'normality' when the body is marginalised in consciousness, taken for granted and minimally intrusive. It is 'absent' in the sense that the individual can act in the world without fear that the body will be the source of serious discomfort, fail to function or betray the self: body and self exist in a state of comparative harmony precisely because the body is, to all intents and purposes, functioning in ways which we usually describe as 'normal'.

Williams's second condition of embodiment is dualism, or the alienation of the body from the self. This occurs when bodies encounter some form of physical resistance. The absent body (Leder 1990), or the body which has been taken for granted, makes its presence felt when illness or disability occur and individual awareness of this biological change forces a sense of separation of self from body. The body no longer functions effortlessly to express the self and a pre-existing experience of harmony is dissipated. The body intrudes on consciousness because it no longer functions painlessly or smoothly and can no longer, as may happen in later life, be ignored or treated as if it is 'absent'.

It is, of course, in later life that the question of the permanence or reversibility of biological change becomes significant, and comparisons between illness and ageing assume a particular urgency. In the biomedical model of human ageing, Williams's third state of embodiment, the struggle to return to the first condition of the taken-for-granted body, is restricted by biological limits to recovery and recuperation. In the constructionist model efforts are made (sometimes on a combative scale as we see in the discussion of Kitwood and Gullette below) to mediate the influence of biology by introducing into the equation the constructionist influences of social interaction and culture. A good example of what may develop into a contest between exponents of the biomedical model and the social constructionist perspective can be found in Kitwood's interactionist analysis of Alzheimer's Disease (1998). In his view, the fact that Alzheimer's Disease is a biomedical reality does not alter the overarching social reality of the construction of personhood through everyday interaction and the potential for sustaining through collective support the individual identity of even the most confused and mentally impaired sufferer. For Kitwood the biomedical model of dementia is morally and socially impoverished. It is 'absurdly reductionist to suggest, as some have done, that "everything in the end comes down to what is going on in individual brain cells"' (1998: 41) and a gross betrayal of our knowledge of the social construction of individual personhood to fail to engage with the 'experiential frame of another person' (*ibid.*: 71).

Williams's threefold sociological model of the vicissitudes of embodiment is indebted to contemporary debates about the interplay between body, self and society in late modernity. As a reflexive model it offers a useful conceptual framework within which to work towards an interactive processual perspective on ageing and decline. Ageing can thus be conceptualised as a process of exchange which crucially includes, as Coupland, *et al.* (1991) have argued in their discursive analyses, the social construction of 'elderliness' in conversations between younger and older women. They clearly demonstrate that the close observation of these exchanges shows that an older person is not *uniformally* old or not old, 'rather, she self-reflects and self projects in and out of the category, aligning herself momentarily with the "old" in respect of some currently salient, desired (or at least tolerated) trait, and then setting herself outside the same group in relation to some other criterion' (*ibid.*: 68). The experience of ageing therefore involves complex movements between categories of age-related social activity depending upon the contexts within which individuals in different age groups interact. It is a matter of social expectations as well as biology. Ethnographic research into the ways in which individuals and groups negotiate the meaning of the ageing process also confirms that ageing is not a terminally invariable condition resulting from physical changes such as the onset of arthritis or alterations in mental function such as memory loss, but an ambiguous and fluctuating process whereby personal identification with the category 'old' varies according to situation, time, and the quality and structure of forms of social interaction. The problem is that there is a tendency to impose the label 'decline' on the known diversity of individual experiences in later life and it this tendency that is the subject of Gullette's radical constructionist analysis of the tensions between biomedical and cultural models of the ageing process.

'Declining to decline'

Margaret Morganroth Gullette is one of the most vigorous and theoretically integrated exponents of the argument that ageing as decline is culturally constructed. The central concern of her work (1988; 1993; 1997; 1998) is a literary and sociological analysis of the processes at work in the social construction of biological ageing as personal and social decline. Her critique begins with the fundamental question of the nature of the boundaries between the ages and stages of life: in other words, how is it possible for us to 'enter' into old age? The concept of life as 'naturally' divided into a linear sequence of 'ages' and 'stages' is deeply embedded in western culture and it is not uncommon to hear references to old age as a condition one enters at a particular point in an inescapable process of decline. In the discipline of social gerontology, as a brief inspection of any textbook reveals (see, for example, Bond *et al.*, 1993), a considerable amount of time and effort has been devoted to the question of the nature of the transition into old age. Biographies of famous people who have become older are another significant source of evidence of this convention, which is often indicated by the designation 'in old age'. One of many examples is a photograph in Jan Marsh's biography of Jane Morris, the widow of the English artist William Morris, which appears above the description: 'Janey *in* old age' (1986: 265, emphasis added). In her memoir of her father's final years in residential care the novelist and biographer Margaret Forster refers to him 'in his old age ... ' (1998: 217). The prevalence of this discursive practice suggests that old age is conceptualised as a physical condition that has an entrance: a finite state of physical being, embodied in both time and space.

The question of 'entrance', therefore, is closely bound up with the idea that old age has an objective biologically grounded existence. In this model, middle age is usually defined as the stage of life when we first become aware of physical deterioration or decline and the finite biological nature of our existence. But the problem with this interpretation of middle age as the point at which ageing into old age begins is the fact that the discursive practice of defining and describing ageing is closely interwoven with *prescription*. A range of culturally prescribed assumptions and expectations around ageing influence an apparently objective analysis of the ageing process. Gullette's criticism of the concept of entrance into old age is that it is a trope dependent 'on accepting the positivist claim of age ideology: that there's a real category of being there, separable from earlier stages or age classes and discontinuous from continuous processes as well' (1997: 159). Entrance is a structural metaphor which generates a specific psychological orientation to ageing that includes a negative set of emotions including regret, a sense of loss, of time passing and of life coming to an end. In this culturally prescribed context, middle age is conventionalised as a period of ageing into old age when it is considered 'normal' for each individual to become increasingly preoccupied with the body and its vicissitudes. As the example from the photograph with caption 'Janey in old age' (Marsh, 1986: 265) shows, changes in the external appearance of the body (in this example, the hair, face, dress and bodily posture) are significant markers of the 'entrance'.

For Gullette 'entrance' is a culturally constructed expectation, the point at which the inevitable process of decline begins: the beginning of being 'in' old age. But, although the origins of decline can be sociologically located in external forms of social organisation and discourse, the master narrative of ageing invariably defines the process as biological and therefore 'naturally' and 'normally' inevitable. When we describe any individual as 'in' old age we dispense with the need to question the presumption of ageing further and to consider alternative forms of explanation. The popular cliché, 'It's my age' is an accepted form of words foreclosing the need for any further discussion.

Gullette's first book, *Safe at Last in the Middle Years*, an exercise in literary gerontology, pursues the argument that 'the decline theory of life' (1988: xviii) is not grounded in a predetermined biological reality but is a master narrative with a demonstrable cultural history. The decline view, as expressed in both non-fictional and fictional western writing, puts the reader in the place of victim of the inevitable ageing process. Drawing on examples from English and American literature she describes the years 1910–1935 as a significant period in the construction of a decline narrative; a defining moment in western culture when there is ample evidence that 'Deficiency and disease were becoming the standard metaphors for normal ageing' (1988: 23). She identifies evidence during this period of a departure from the traditional ages-and-stages model of the lifecourse, as the onset of ageing (midlife) was relocated to an earlier point than previously. As the result of changes in age consciousness, produced by the transformation of socio-economic life, a preoccupation with middle age became more urgent and more central to personal identity. And this concern was culturally elaborated through an interplay of medical (geriatric medicine), gerontological (concerned with the emerging study of social and psychological aspects of ageing), and fictional works. Under, for example, the influence of the new hormone theories of specialists such as the American expert G. Stanley Hall, an 'imaginary life course' (Gullette, 1988: 27) was created in literary culture for both men and women: 'One of the most striking phenomena of the new century is that literature ... began with some frequency to age its main characters into the middle years and beyond ... Suddenly a host of characters in their forties or in some vague middle age began to appear and simultaneously decay' (*ibid.*). Thus a connection was made in the public imagination between chronological age and decline in strength, energy, self-control, physical confidence and creativity. Writers of fiction, says Gullette, gave 'subjective content to the otherwise empty rhetoric of the ageing manuals' (1988: 28) and the fear of ageing was exaggerated in the literature of the time beyond the range of everyday experience. As she wryly notes in her essay, 'Creativity, Ageing, Gender', 'The amount of desperation about ageing that was circulating in the culture went far beyond what any writer could personally have experienced of loss through the processes of age alone' (1993: 29). In this cultural climate it becomes increasingly difficult to conjure up positive images of middle age and later life. The biological changes associated with chronological ageing are interpreted within a powerfully negative and pessimistic frame of reference.

But the ageing body/aged by culture question is complex and subtle and Gullette's sustained critique of the hegemony of the master status of a culture in which the narrative of decline is dominant should not be taken to mean that biological ageing is marginalised as merely a socially constructed cultural artefact. The body is real enough to Gullette, who includes references to some of her own bodily problems (for example osteoarthritis) in the autobiographical pages of *Declining to Decline* (1997). As a constructionist, Gullette's central argument is that a significant distinction can be made between the biological body which grows older and is subject to pain, illness and disability and the 'traditional decline view' (1988: xiii) where decline is seen as the unifying and exclusive characteristic of the ageing process. Gullette's constructionism is one that focuses on the *connections* we make between the biological, the psychological and the social which are culturally prescribed and therefore open to revision and change. The decline narrative or the story we tell about ageing (Hepworth, 2000) is a device for establishing connections between a number of essentially diverse and disparate biological processes (she cites tooth decay and loss, the menopause, her own menopause) in order to construct what is essentially an imaginary story of comprehensive and universal decline. It is not, therefore, that biological decline in old age is a figment of the western imagination; it is the connections we make that are fictions and as such the conscious/unconscious reflections of a dominant ideology. Ageing as a narrative provides us with a wide range of spurious links between the variable biological changes that take place as the body changes (variably, internally – function and 'absence', and externally – appearance) and the result is a series of stereotyped images of what it means to be an old person. A good example is the assumption, subtly researched, for example, by Coupland *et al.* (1991), that older people are excessively preoccupied with their health, well-being, mobility, and lifestyle as they grow older. In Gullette's words, deterioration is 'a cultural label with a complicated history' (1997: 157).

The connections between the biological, psychological and social aspects of ageing are established through a process of learning to associate the changes taking place in the body with the onset of decline. The entrance to old age via middle age is made through the cultivation of the 'age gaze', a learned perceptual frame of self-labelling as an ageing individual, 'by learning appropriate practices and a set of knowledges guiding the age gaze. That gaze sweeps over our imperceptibly changing anatomy and decides *when* to speak, negatively of "changed" looks' (*ibid.*: 169). These shared practices effectively constrain the diversity of experiences of middle and later life within the procrustean bed of a 'universal wholly biological process' (*ibid.*: 212). Acceptance of the belief that ageing is essentially a process of biological decline and appropriate self-labelling as 'old' submerges the multiplicity of social identities that help constitute the individuality of each person beneath a uniform and ageist stereotype (references to multiplicity can be compared with Stephen Katz's Foucauldian argument that ageing is now 'polysemic' [1996: 40]). For Gullette, identity, which is a category of difference, is submerged by 'age', a category of similarity and uniformity. Conformity of the individual older person (who subjectively experiences difference) to expectations of 'age-identity' (the external social category of 'ageing') transforms the subject into a victim of mid-life: a process of subordination not to biology but to a cultural interpretation of biology and the repression of diversity.

Whilst this universal plot is deeply gendered and there are significant differences between the experiences of women and men, Gullette, in common with a number of other analysts (Benson, 1997; Featherstone and Hepworth, 1998b), also detects evidence of gender convergence in mid-life. As the most significant biological variable in mid-life, the menopause is the quintessential example of a physical change that is regarded as symptomatic of an inevitable biological decline in function. But it is because many of the negative experiences of the menopause are now understood as the product of the strong cultural association of desirable feminity with reproductive function that changes in the position of women in society are also altering male perceptions and experience of middle age. If in the past men, and in particular socially advantaged men, were protected by the differential balance of power from the negative associations of mid-life and were able to present male middle age as the highpoint of 'maturity', in more recent times this traditional 'male immunity to midlife ageing' is being eroded, 'bringing men psychologically closer to the situation that women are supposed to experience at midlife' (Featherstone and Hepworth, 1998b: 161). In other words, the experience of the menopause as decline is causally connected with the degree of social status that is conferred on older women and men: biological change is not necessarily decline.

Whilst contemporary consumer culture has fostered more positive images of life after 50 for those with sufficient income and resources to participate in the emerging midlifestyles (Hepworth and Featherstone, 1982; Featherstone and Hepworth, 1998b), middle age for thousands of men is becoming increasingly associated with downward social mobility. In Gullette's (1998) view, the decline narrative of middle age is now much more prevalent partly as a result of discrimination against middle-aged men in the field of employment. Amongst the negative factors at work she includes the detrimental effects of redundancy on incomes at midlife and a decline in the social status of men whose former career expectations included steady enhancement into maturity. One problem is that privileged middle-class professional men, who in the past tended to epitomise a gendered vision of midlife as a peak period of prosperity (portraits of prosperous professionals and entrepreneurs with well-fed physical proportions come to mind), are now exposed to the insecurity and unemployment that result from restructuring the economy and the reduction in opportunities for 'jobs for life'. Redundancy and early retirement reinforce the biologistic conception of midlife as the 'entrance' into a declining later life. The well-fed middle-aged male body is no longer a public sign of consolidated achievement and security; the 'paunch' or 'corporation' of the past can no longer be displayed without the risk of censure and threat to self-confidence and is now regarded as evidence of potential weakness and the risk of impending decline.

This shift in the balance of power also has the potential for removing men from the protective care of women who in the past, Gullette argues, 'were taught to feel older but not to notice men feeling older' (1997: 151). Changes in the socio-economic status of men in the 50+ age range have the effect of bringing their emotions closer to the surface, thus making it more likely that they will seek new forms of emotional expression as they grow older. The male menopause will, Gullette predicts, follow the history of the construction of the menopause, beginning amongst the more socially advantaged, where codes of perfection are stricter, competition keener and the fear of failure is greater (Featherstone and Hepworth, 1998b). A key feature is the increasing experience amongst men of 'midlife helplessness': 'In a story of midlife helplessness, the climacteric will soon loom much larger. They'll teach men that *their* ageing results from a hormone deficiency disease and that it can be cured by buying chemicals or implants' (1997: 146). There will be a generalisation of the 'midlife crisis' as it diffuses down the social register and changes from the special condition of a few to become 'somehow both pathological and universal, linked to self-loathing and sexual dysfunction' (1997: 147). One is immediately reminded of the ramifications of the impact of the promotion of Viagra for sexual impotency in later life: a significant example of the tendency of the dominant biological model of ageing is to medicalise mid- and later life.

In Gullette's work the balance between ageing bodies and a culture that ages epitomises the struggle between biological and socially constructed models of ageing where the former defines ageing negatively as decline and the latter holds out the promise of creating positive discourses of ageing which celebrate and promote the ideology of a positive diversity of human identities in later life. In the process of positive resistance to biologically grounded narratives the concept of decline is detached from ageing and replaced by a concept of change that creates space for personal self-assertion and growth. Gullette's positive narrative does not end 'in' old age because the notion of later life as a terminus will have been completely deconstructed. Once sociological analysis makes it possible to identify the social forces at work in the construction and maintenance of the concept of decline; the imaginary nature of a lifecourse as a one-way process becomes clear. Once it is clear that the causal connections between the biological, psychological and social aspects of ageing are narrative connections, then defensible grounds for optimism about the future of later life emerge. In Gullette's words: 'The idea that we might escape being aged by culture is breathtaking' (1997: 18). and the desire is fostered to discard the 'standard social meaning' of the ageing body and 'hold tight to a complex idiosyncratic narrative of age identity' (*ibid.*).

Gullette's advocacy of the potential of liberation from the decline narrative if not from the finitude of the body has no place for facile optimism. Her conception of the cultural space which may be created to produce a diversity of positive discourses of mid- and later life is counterbalanced by an empirically grounded awareness of the resilience of the discourse of decline. Indeed, the whole key to Gullette's analysis is the knowledge that the decline model always lives to fight another day and the watchword must be constant vigilance.

Thus her studies of the intersections between creativity, ageing, and gender since the early twentieth century show how the decline model exists alongside evidence of efforts to construct a 'new ideology of ageing ... in the "midlife progress novel"' (1988: xii). The mid-life progress novel imagines mid-life as a time for personal reassessment and self-realisation. Mid-life is not the point of entry to decline but an opportunity for positive change experienced as renewal; as such this form of fiction presents its readers with new heroes and heroines of the middle years. In *Safe at Last in the Middle Years* these heroes and heroines share the defining characteristic of 'resistances, strengths, or sly timely weaknesses, ingenious mental feints' (1988: xiv). Gullette's scholarly literary analysis of the social construction of midlife shows how each of her selected authors 'came to produce one or a few midlife progress narratives' (1988: xxvii); a process described as 'a private adventure in *changing one's genre*' (1988: xxviii). The authors she selects to trace the emergence of positive images of mid-life are: John Updike's novels, in particular his 'Rabbit' series; Margaret Drabble, including *Jerusalem The Golden*, *The Middle Ground* and *The Ice Age*; Anne Tyler, including *Earthly Possessions*, *Celestial Navigation* and *The Clock Winder*; and Saul Bellow, including *Humbolt's Gift* and *Seize The Day*. Their literary engagement with midlife confronts the widespread assumption that creativity in general, and literary creativity in particular, begins to decline during the middle years. It provides readers with evidence of 'an array of models of how to become in the middle years' (Gullette, 1988: xvi). Authors of this kind of fiction not only offer their reading public an alternative to the decline narrative of midlife but also refute in the act of creative writing the assumption that literary creativity is undermined by age. The key is identification with the 'psychological direction of the genre' which enables each individual reader to construct his or her own version of the story (*ibid.*: xvi). 'This identification is the fundamental *condition of possibility*' (*ibid.*: xvi).

The reason for the resilience of the decline model is the appeal it makes to realism. For Gullette the difficulty with the decline narrative is that it poses as the ultimate biomedical reality of the lifecourse. In the fictional and non-fictional literature of ageing the point of connection with personal feelings has often been through the powerful idea of the inevitability of decay and consequently disillusionment with life. At work here is what Gullette describes as the 'essentialist illusion' (1988: 20). The essentialist illusion blames biological ageing for all the negative experiences of later life, including the decline in literary creativity. It can be added that so pervasive is this view that those in the creative arts who apparently 'triumph' over the decline essentially associated with later life are regarded as unusually heroic. Spectacular examples include the artists Rembrandt, Renoir and, more recently, Picasso, and the film-star and singer Marlene Dietrich. Their performances, in some respects not unlike those of lesser mortals who are seen as 'good for their age', are often described in those tones of awe and wonder that only serve to reinforce the commonsensical belief that decline is 'normal'. In effect such survivors of the 'normal' ageing process simply postpone their entrance into old age. As heroes and heroines of ageing they become, as Goffman (1968) has observed of celebrities of physical disability, not representatives of a wider population but exceptions to the rule.

The resolution of the shifting balance of power between positive/negative and change/diversity/decline constructions of ageing may be found, according to Gullette, in the vision of the 'portmanteau' or postmodern self (1997: 220). Because the self is not a biological entity but a narrative construct it is possible to explore the rich variety of ways in which biological changes can be accommodated in any personal life story. The master narrative of decline describes a single self going through a linear trajectory whilst the portmanteau self is 'an active concept of ageing as self-narrated experience, the conscious, ongoing story of one's age identity' (1997: 220). Because decline is constructed as a narrative, the route of escape cannot be *into* the body modified, for example, through cosmetic surgery, or the body of the cyborg – part biology, part technology (Leng, 1996) – but into an alternative liberated narrative of the self. The body is thus 'minimal' (Gullette, 1997: 221) because in Gullette's analyis the decline associated with ageing is primarily an ideological construct and as such can be changed by human action. In this sense ageing as decline is not biological but a cultural script which draws on interpretations of biological reality to justify the decline. For this reason Gullette considers techniques of body modification designed to combat the physical signs of ageing (for example, cosmetic surgery, HRT) to be grounded in a nostalgic view of the body. Cosmetic surgery and HRT both involve attempts (a) to stop the clock and remain in the present or (b) to return to the past of one's younger days: an interesting irony in a society that is supposedly future-oriented (see Justine Coupland's chapter in this volume). In contrast, Gullette's work is a sustained effort to *imagine* a positively ageing self: a postmodern self characterised by a multiplicity of narratives that transcend the biological frame.

And yet, for all the vigorous constructionism in this account, the problem of the ageing body is not completely resolved. In *Safe at Last in the Middle Years* Gullette finds hope in the 'midlife progress narrative' which requires 'readers willing to identify with adult protagonists who are not ultimately haunted by their ageing bodies' (1988: xx). And yet, as she observes in *Declining to Decline*, human beings 'do not have to love every aspect of their "me" to value their identity ... In fact, the people likely to gain most are those who dislike the parts of self that have come to them labelled as "bodily" and "ageing"' (1997: 216). It is at this point that the mask of ageing (Featherstone and Hepworth, 1991) emerges from the shadows to take up a more central position in the analysis of the relationship between the ageing body, and the self. For one of the difficulties with the ageing body, as Leder (1990) and Williams (1996) have shown, is that it is remarkably obdurate and it tends to intrude into subjective and social life. As all empirical research on ageing into old age repeatedly shows, the body in later life just will not go away: it cannot under all circumstances be dissolved into an interplay of postmodern discourses.

At the same time, there remains a world of difference between a negative acceptance of stereotypes of ageing as decline and efforts to make positive and radical reconstructions of images of ageing. Because ageist stereotypes are legitimised by a concept of decline as an inevitable biologically determined point of closure, the struggle may seem superficial and destined for ultimate failure. But for Gullette it is the acceptance of the decline narrative in its various forms (including the modification of the external appearance of the body) that is superficial and negative. Her argument is that the decline narrative is only one amongst a choice of several narratives of ageing – alternatives have been emerging, for example, for some years in literary culture. Confronting the paradox of the ageing body, Gullette accentuates the notion of the core self which she defines as a narrative of the persistence of the self engaged in a lifelong struggle to maintain individual integrity. In her view the time is now ripe for a more positive integration of the biological, psychological and social processes of ageing. Integrative action of this order does not prioritise one period of the lifecourse (often, of course, the values associated with the appearance of youth) but imagines and experiences growing older as the cultivation of a continuous life-story: a journey of the self into the future rather than a nostalgic fixation on an identity that has been buried somewhere in the past with the body of a previous identity.

Acknowledgement

An earlier version of the discussion of the work of Margaret Morganroth Gullette was published in M. Hepworth 'In Defiance of An Ageing Culture' in *Ageing and Society* 19 (1999): 139–48. Cambridge: Cambridge University Press. The author and publisher gratefully acknowledge the permission of Cambridge University Press to quote extensively from this chapter.

References

Bendelow, G. and Williams, S. (1995) 'Pain and the Mind-Body Dualism: A Sociological Approach', *Body & Society* 1 (2): 83–103.

Benson, J. (1997) *Prime Time: A History of the Middle Aged in Twentieth-century Britain*. London and New York: Longman.

Bond, J., Coleman, P. and Peace, S. (1993) *Ageing in Society: an Introduction to Social Gerontology* (2nd edn). London: Sage.

Bytheway, B. (1985) *The Later Part of Life: a Study of the Concept of Old Age*. University College of Swansea, School of Social Studies: Occasional Paper No 10.

Bytheway, B. (1997) 'Talking About Age: the Theoretical Basis of Social Gerontology'. In A. Jamieson, S. Harper and C. Victor (eds) *Critical Approaches to Ageing and Later Life*. Buckingham: Open University Press.

Cole, T.R. (1992) *The Journey of Life: a Cultural History of Ageing in America*. Cambridge, New York: Cambridge University Press.

Coupland, N., Coupland, J. and Giles, H. (1991) *Language, Society and the Elderly: Discourse, Identity and Ageing.* Oxford, UK and Cambridge, MA: Blackwell.

Featherstone, M. and Hepworth, M. (1991) 'The Mask of Ageing and the Postmodern Life Course'. In M. Featherstone, M. Hepworth and B.S. Turner (eds) *The Body: Social Process and Cultural Theory.* London: Sage.

Featherstone, M. and Hepworth, M. (1998a) 'Ageing, the Lifecourse and the Sociology of Embodiment'. In G. Scambler and P. Higgs (eds) *Modernity, Medicine and Health: Medical Sociology Towards 2000.* London and New York: Routledge.

Featherstone, M. and Hepworth, M. (1998b) 'The Male Menopause: Lay Accounts and the Cultural Reconstruction of Midlife'. In S. Nettleton and J. Watson (eds) *The Body in Everyday Life.* London and New York: Routledge.

Forster, M. (1998) *Precious Lives.* London: Chatto & Windus.

Frank, A. (1996) 'Reconciliatory Alchemy: Bodies Narratives and Power', *Body and Society* 2 (3): 53–71.

Goffman, E. (1968) *Stigma: Notes on the Management of Spoiled Identity.* Harmondsworth: Penguin.

Gubrium, J.F. (1986) *Oldtimers and Alzheimer's: the Descriptive Organisation of Senility.* Greenwich, CT/London: JAI Press.

Gullette, M.M. (1988) *Safe at Last in the Middle Years, the Invention of the Midlife Progress Novel: Saul Bellow, Margaret Drabble, Anne Tyler, and John Updike.* Berkeley, Los Angeles and London: University of California Press.

Gullette, M.M. (1993) 'Creativity, Ageing, Gender: a Study in their Intersections, 1910–1935'. In A.M. Wyatt Brown and J. Rossen (eds) *Ageing and Gender in Literature: Studies in Creativity.* Charlottesville and London: University Press of Virginia.

Gullette, M.M. (1997) *Declining to Decline: Cultural Combat and the Politics of the Midlife.* Charlottesville and London: University Press of Virginia.

Gullette, M.M. (1998) 'The Politics of Middle Ageism'. *New Political Science* 20 (3): 263–82.

Hepworth, M. (2000) *Stories of Ageing.* Buckingham: Open University Press.

Hepworth, M. and Featherstone, M. (1982) *Surviving Middle Age.* Oxford: Basil Blackwell.

Katz, S. (1996) *Disciplining Old age: the Formation of Gerontological Knowledge.* Charlottesville and London: University Press of Virginia.

Kitwood, T. (1998) *Dementia Reconsidered: the Person Comes First.* Buckingham: Open University Press.

Leder, D. (1990) *The Absent Body.* Chicago: University of Chicago Press.

Leng, K.W. (1996) 'On Menopause and Cyborgs: Or, Towards a Feminist Cyborg Politics of Menopause'. *Body & Society* 2 (3) 33–52.

Marsh, J. (1986) *Jane and May Morris: A Biographical Study 1839–1938.* London and New York: Pandora.

Nuland, S.B. (1997) *How We Die.* London: Vintage.

Toombs, S. Kay. (1993) *The Meaning of Illness: a Phenomenological Account of the Different Perspectives of Physician and Patient.* Dordrecht: Kluwer.

Williams, S. (1996) 'The Vicissitudes of Embodiment Across the Chronic Illness Trajectory'. *Body and Society* 2 (2): 23–47.

Woodward, K. (1991) *Ageing and its Discontents: Freud and Other Fictions.* Bloomington and Indianapolis: Indiana University Press.

6
Tales of Outrage and the Everyday: Fear of Crime and Bodies at Risk

Marian Tulloch and John Tulloch

A couple of years ago, in the small community of Snowtown in South Australia, police announced the discovery in a disused bank vault of a number of bodies decomposing in drums of acid. The find created great media and public interest, particularly as further bodies were located, in what was rapidly labelled Australia's worst serial killing. Yet, despite the rather ghoulish fascination, the response to the case evinced none of the wave of emotion, indignation and demand for public action that accompanied the massacre at Port Arthur, Tasmania, some years earlier. It appears not all bodies are equal, nor do their deaths generate the same level of fear and anxiety about the risk of violent crime. These two multiple killings present contrasting moral tales, each disclosing the frames through which the media and the public interpret and react to violence. The chapter uses the concept of outrage to explore how bodies, and in particular female bodies, are constructed as sites of risk and to suggest how such representations can be challenged.

Outrage, a term that describes an emotional yet action-oriented response to events, has been applied in the field of environmental risk communication to explain why public reaction and risk perception are often at variance with expert hazard assessment (Sandman, 1987a). The factors identified as influencing outrage can be consolidated under the broad categories of impact, personal control and moral relevance. Outrage is greatest when events are exotic, memorable, temporally and geographically focused, with perceived dreadful consequences, when they are involuntary and controlled by 'the system', and when they are morally relevant. While Sandman's construction of outrage was particularly developed to understand community responses to environmental risk, it can also illuminate media and community response to crimes of violence. Certainly the Port Arthur killings were dread-provoking in their savagery and characterised by a temporally and geographically focused exotic location, with random and unfairly targeted victims. English (1991) has argued that it is the latter moral factor, including victims' rights to be protected by adequate risk management, that is most important in explaining levels of outrage. High outrage is dependent on a worthy victim whose rights are violated, an agent with perceived high level of moral responsibility for the prevention of risk and a perceived failure to manage that risk. Thus, while horrific crimes can focus the community anger against the perpetrator, community outrage is most likely to result from the failure of public authorities to protect citizens deemed worthy of protection. Media coverage of the Snowtown and Port Arthur murders presents moral tales. At Port Arthur (as at Dunblane) worthy citizens including children, for whom the community has a special duty of care, became random victims of society's lax approach to gun control. By contrast, at Snowtown the victims from a socio-economically disadvantaged area were members of a socially marginal group which, according to an early news conference, 'preyed upon itself' (a reference, it later emerged, to the claim that social security fraud motivated the killings). The first victim was labelled 'a known paedophile'. On initial information, the case presented neither worthy victims nor evidence of a failure of societal risk management.

The media and the female body at risk

The media deal in outrage and thus set public agendas about the threat of crime. Their focus is on the dramatic, unusual, vicious crime; accounts of violence against women place emphasis on random sexually motivated attacks by unknown assailants in public space. By focusing on crimes that engender public reaction, the unusual and atypical is privileged over the everyday and commonplace. This poses the question as to whether these powerful tales, often characterised as media sensationalism, determine the way that people, and women in particular, understand the risk of criminal violence and the construction of worthy victims. Does the media create in women an 'unrealistically' high fear of crime?

From a feminist perspective, Weaver *et al.* (2000) argue that media coverage of violence against women is both a product and a reinforcement of a patriarchal system of female subordination. The media focus on public sexual violence constructs 'the female body as a site of risk' and leads to women being irrationally fearful in public space while ignoring the much greater risks of private violence. Their argument is worth detailed consideration because it provides specific evidence of how women respond to media portrayals of violence in constructing a personal understanding of risk. They draw on qualitative focus group data from the Schlesinger *et al.* (1992) *Women Viewing Violence* study to argue that series like *America's Most Wanted* and *Crimewatch UK* encourage women to anticipate danger, and to inhibit their activities outside the home as a way to avoid it. Given that many of the respondents had experience of domestic violence committed against them by male intimates, it was seen as surprising that women systematically associated public spaces (particularly at night) with personal risk, and, when they did speak of fears of violent attacks in their homes, also tended to associate these risks with male strangers. In particular, the researchers drew on women's responses to a *Crimewatch* hitch-hiking item to argue that the 'unnecessary risk' assessment of hitch-hiking by most women indicated the way in which women negotiate their everyday lives by privileging a gendered distinction between public and private spaces. Drawing on feminist social geographers' emphasis that severe restrictions on women's mobility in public spaces have been crucial to the perpetuation of their subordination in Western societies, Weaver *et al.* observe that 'this further demonstrates the ways in which patriarchal assumptions, through the particular types of discursive strategies used in crime reporting, encourage women to "adopt false assumptions about their security when in places falsely deemed safe for women, such as the home"' (Valentine, 1989:385).

Secondly, Weaver *et al.* discuss the ideological role of the media more generally in shaping women's sense of risks when they enter public spaces. Drawing on Carter's own analysis of the British tabloid press (as well as other media-related content analysis), they point out that there is a systematic over-representation of the threat posed by male strangers in relation to their officially recorded occurrence. Carter's work showed that while Home Office figures indicated that only 13 per cent of female victims were killed by a male stranger, over 40 per cent of all news on sexual violence in British tabloids fell within this category. Further, the language journalists recurrently use renders news reports of sexual violence unthreatening to 'normal' men by a focus on men whose violence is deemed to be *excessive* and female victims whose suffering is deemed to be *undeserved* (namely women who by dress and demeanour do not transgress the spatial and ideological boundaries of patriarchal definitions of femininity). 'Thus, labels like "monster", "fiend" and "animal" are employed to refer to some offenders in order to individualise and personalise the violence. The use of such terms invites the reader to divert blame away from ... a patriarchal system which perpetuates structural gender inequalities based on the economic, social and cultural subordination of women' (Weaver *et al.*, 2000). Occupational ideologies within journalism here collude with a patriarchal 'consensual worldview' to condemn violence against 'good' women and girls, and to caution those who are irresponsible in taking 'unreasonable' risks (that is those who reject their protected space within 'safe' domesticity). The construction of public tales of crimes against women positions them within a crime prevention discourse that distorts real risks and focuses on female responsibility for self-protection while the responsibility of males for their own violence is ignored (Stanko, 1996). Moreover, by pathologising the violent stranger as a 'monster', the gendered nature of these attacks and the normalcy of male violence are obscured.

Thirdly, Weaver *et al.* draw on Stanko's and other researchers' work on fear of crime, specifically on the state's encouragement of women to avoid the lurking male menace – how to travel ('with petrol in your car'), how to dress, how to walk, how to talk, how to appear assertive and in control of their modern lives. Weaver *et al.* argue that crime prevention discourses largely ignore the main risks to women (which are within domesticity), targeting the potential danger to women in public environments. As the researchers argue, according to the media 'Only "beasts" hurt women. Yet we now know that most violence against women is perpetrated by "nice guys", not "beasts".' This continuing media agenda encourages the ongoing finding that women report fear of crime at three times the level of men, even though their recorded risk of personal violence (especially assault) is lower than men's according to official sources. It is this broad societal/media consensus, worked through female socialisation from a very early age, that explains why, 'when one asks women about danger, their fears translate into concerns about the dangers lurking in the physical environment: parking lots, public stairwells, and public transit, for instance, are typically named by women as dangerous places in community safety audits' (Weaver *et al.*, 2000: 182).

Weaver *et al.* conclude that media reports of sexual violence are 'shaped by an ideology of the "respectable" (domesticised, privatised) woman who adheres to traditional expectations for women under any patriarchal regime. Home, family and sexual propriety are expected to shield women from harm' (Weaver *et al.*, 2000: 182). By adopting a wide range of everyday, mundane routines in public places to avoid the violation of sexual integrity, women are acknowledging the potential of sexual violence 'as a core component of their *being female*' (Weaver *et al.*, 2000: 182). Women are thus policing themselves in public environments, using more safety precautions than men. The 'media clearly play a key role in socialising women to accept their subordinate status by way of constructing the female body as a site of risk' (*ibid*: 183).

However, while contributing to the understanding of the gendered public discourse about crime and violence, Weaver *et al.*'s argument is in danger of itself constructing women as passive and homogeneous in their responses to the media and criminal threat; not all women are afraid nor are all men fearless (Gilchrist *et al.*, 1998). The argument that women wrongly fear violence in public and ignore private risk has the potential to recreate the 'irrational' woman who greatly over-estimates risk in public places, thus becoming a media dupe who has 'bought into' patriarchal explanations (Weaver *et al.*, 2000). In this chapter, we want to draw attention to our reservations about this, derived both from current media theory and from our own large-scale fear of crime research in Australia. Furthermore, we want to argue that a concept of outrage mobilised by a rights rather than a risk discourse represents a way of looking more strategically and less monolithically at the construction of narratives of crime in public debate. The implications of this alternative approach enable the creation of fissures and counter-definitions in the moral tales that circulate in public discourse and may help mobilise public policy.

'The female body at risk' and the current state of media theory

The impact on women of media representation of crime needs to be set in the context of current debates in media/audience theory. Weaver *et al.*'s approach to the effects of the media tends to resurrect older, some would say 'outmoded', notions of the passive viewer. In our view, though, Weaver *et al.* (2000) have made a valuable intervention into current media audience discussion and the area of media and fear of crime specifically. They rightly complain that the insights of feminist commentators into the role of the media in women's fear of crime have been ignored not only by public commentators from state agencies but also by academic media theorists. The part played by the media in socially constructing gendered spaces within and between public and private environments has been inadequately theorised. There are, we think, at least two main reasons for this lack of interest among news media researchers. First, the 'ideological effect' emphasis of Weaver *et al.*'s piece, while strong in media studies during the 1970s, weakened substantially in the 1980s where a new emphasis on the 'active audience' tended to ignore the mass media's power and effectivity. In particular, the focus on women's pleasures in fictional forms (Ang, 1985; 1996) tended to take attention away from women's fears about risk as conveyed by the media (which is why we regard Schlesinger *et al.*'s (1992) *Women Viewing Violence* as an important counter to this trend). Secondly, the recent interest among sociologists such as Beck, Giddens and Wynne on the 'risk society', while *assuming* a large place for the media, has been very remiss in not providing theories about the processes through which this media 'effect' occurs. The chapter by Weaver *et al.* is welcome in both these areas: redirecting our attention to important feminist work around 'place', 'space' and media representation; and in at least gesturing in the direction of the need to flesh out 'risk' approaches to women, the body and news media via theories of journalistic organisational values, narrativisation and discourse.

This argument is taken further in the introduction to the book in which the Weaver *et al.* piece appears (Allan *et al.*, 2000). Here the editors argue for the need to examine the 'fissures' that occur between 'expert' consensus and audience response to the media. It may be, they say, at this point in the relationship between media and audiences that:

> the antagonisms between those who produce risk definitions and those who consume them are at their most apparent ... [I]t is ... important to keep in mind that at the same time the media are playing a crucial role in sustaining the imperatives of 'expert' risk assessment, they are also creating spaces, albeit under severe constraints, for counter-definitions to emerge ... This is to suggest, then, that the identification of slips, fissures, silences and gaps in media reporting need to be accompanied by a search for alternatives.
>
> (*Ibid.*: 14)

In fact potential fissures are evident in the analysis of the hitch-hiking story that Weaver *et al.* present. Although many respondents accept the construction of hitch-hiking as risky behaviour, some do not.

Instead they argue that this blames the victim rather than focusing on the perpetrators. In the indignant words of one woman:

> Why should we be the ones to stop hitchhiking? They should be catching the people that murder these people.
>
> (Weaver *et al.*, 2000: 175)

Her outrage is directed not just at the murderers but at 'they' who fail to catch them. Her question represents a shift in discourse about crime from one based on risk to one based on rights. To understand this distinction and its relevance to the concept of outrage a more interactive model of the relation of audience and media text is needed. Within media and cultural studies a new phase of what Pertii Alasuutari (2000) is calling 'third generation' audience studies provides an approach to such analyses. It attempts to synthesise the 'ideological effect' emphasis of the 1970s with the 'active audience' research of the 1980s via empirical research into the 'moral frames' within which both production and reception of media texts are embedded. This chapter will begin to explore 'moral frames' circulating in the media and in everyday interaction by a study of people's talk about criminal threat and the way media and individual everyday experience are interwoven in their tales.

Women, risk and tales of the everyday

To explore how the reading of media messages is negotiated through personal experience and wider informal circuits of communication, this chapter draws on data from our study of fear of crime (Tulloch *et al.*, 1998). Participants talked in focus groups and long interviews about their personal experiences and their reactions to media coverage of crime. For these men and women, the media is just one of a series of interconnected formal and informal circuits of communication contributing to their perception of the threat of criminal violence, a perception inflected in terms of their own experiences and sociocultural location.

In discussions of crime and the media, participants frequently mentioned the programme *Australia's Most Wanted*, the Australian equivalent of *Crimewatch*, one of the shows studied by Weaver *et al.* (2000). The format of the show, presenting real unsolved, often violent crimes, is seen by some viewers as a source of important information but the portrayal of criminals on the loose also generates strong emotional reactions and a heightened sense of vulnerability:

After I watch it, I go to ring Paul up from work or something, and it's like 'go to the window and watch me get into the car'.

[Young female[1]][2]

Such reactions could be interpreted simply as media-induced fear of crime. An approach/avoidance response was a common reaction to this depiction of real Australian crimes:

Because it's real. I don't really want to know about it. *America's Most Wanted* is alright.

[Young female]

Yet the complexity of responses is reflected by one interviewee, drawn to the show but sometimes unable to cope with the emotions it aroused, who recounted her personal experiences as victim of a violent attack in her own home. Like many other female respondents, she spoke of how she attempted to manage television viewing, consciously avoiding material that produced disempowering levels of fear.

Yet taking control of the television may not remove fear. Highlighting the role of the media in creating women's fear of crime in public space may have led to an under-estimation of women's direct sources of information about risk. Reliance on official statistics to assess the level of violence by women has long been criticised by feminists as ignoring much unreported violence, particularly by known assailants. Moreover, women in public space are subjected to a continuum of violence ranging from stares and comments to more overt harassment and violence (Kelly, 1996). Only the more extreme behaviours are reported as crimes but all these actions serve as evidence of potential risk (Tulloch, 2000). Our female respondents discuss issues of agency and bodies at risk in this context of everyday unease and harassment. Young women's accounts of travelling on public transport demonstrate a keen sensitivity to bodily cues. Male gaze, unsolicited comments, unwelcome proximity and touch, signs of alcohol or drug use and other signifiers of deviancy are all taken as cues to potential serious violence. Young women report frequent minor harassment: unwanted attempts at conversations, unwelcome proximity and even 'funny looks' from men. Quite often the men appear drunk or stoned or just 'weird'. These accounts illustrate what Burt and Estep (1981) have described as a process during adolescence in which girls are socialised into a fear of sexual assault through the heightened experience of harassment that leads in turn to self-imposed behavioural constraints.

Although many of these young women claim to be unaffected by the media and to rely on personal experience in assessing risk, the male predator of media headlines appears in their interpretation of the everyday:

> In *Australia's Most Wanted* they always show a picture of the person that you see doing it and you always think it looks like someone you know.
> [Chorus of 'yes']

> And then you think you've seen the person somewhere around so you sort of look around more.
> Yeah, you see him everywhere ...
>
> [Focus group, young females]

As they monitor strange males in public space they are on the lookout for potential threats.

However, this does not imply that the known is equated with safety. Young women's tales of everyday violence – a young male who puts a choke chain round a respondent's neck on the school bus, another who follows a young woman from the bus in order to harass her – carry a more generalised message of threat. Instead of operating with simple distinctions between public and private spheres, known or unknown assailants, young women seem well aware of the threat of assault by males that they know and this fosters a general fear of rape:

> *Interviewer*: When it happened to someone you know, did it make you more worried about your own safety?
> *Respondent* [young female]: With sexual assault it did, because my friend nearly got raped by someone she had known for years and was really close to the family.
> *Respondent* [young female]: When we had the ... self defence thing, he talked about people being jumped on and that sort of thing and I'm paranoid now ...
> [Crime most feared?] I think possibly rape, because we are young women and it's so, it's just awful for that to happen to somebody, that ... man said something like four in ten girls get raped by people they know ...

A tale of a schoolyard rape demonstrates how the unknown assailant can turn out to be known:

Respondent [young female]: I went to school with a girl who was bashed and raped at the back of our school, and we had big school meetings and everything and this guy ended up being from our school.

Interviewer: And how did that make you feel?

Respondent [young female]: Pretty scary. I used to talk to him heaps. And I used to go 'No, no, no, no'. Lucky we didn't go for that little walk.

The dangerous stranger is not passively absorbed from sensational media stories; he is constructed in the tales circulated by these young women that draw both on the media and their everyday experiences. This tale of a schoolmate who is unmasked as a violent rapist was immediately preceded in the focus group discussion by an account of an episode of *Australia's Most Wanted* in which a rapist dressed as a woman had attacked a young girl. The story had added resonance for the group because it occurred in their own town, in a street they knew well. The unmasking of the known as 'other' is always a possibility. Yet everyday tales of sexual violence do not shift the focus from strangers to known men as a source of risk. Rather the everyday threat from fellow students at school, on the bus or at a party reinforces the threat posed by unknown strangers.

Yet, despite the threat of vicious attackers lurking behind the accounts of the everyday, there are also tales that undercut the gulf between the normal male and the deviant attacker. The tension between the 'monstrous' and the everyday is most clearly evident in a woman's tale of a friend raped by a stranger while out walking:

Respondent [female, middle years]: He just kept dragging her back and finally um, finally she fought him and fought him and fought him ... then he raped her and then he said to her 'can I give you a lift home?' And she was sitting there expecting that she would be killed and she just said, because she had you know, seen him and everything, and she said she just sat there and said no, I'll find my own way home and he drove off. Um, it changed; it wasn't a typical ...

Interviewer: Not what you'd expect a rape to be like?

Respondent: No. No. The violence was terrible, but the end bit of it. And then later on, just last year, [my husband] and I were watching a programme on television. It was just a movie, and, but it was a trial for a rape and um, there was something like this that happened in it, that, at the end. It happened in the girl's home and it was someone that she knew, the friend of her flatmate or something, and at the end he sort of said to her 'Can I get you a drink, can I do this'. And the evidence that was given was you know, would a man who has just raped this woman do this? and [my husband] was sitting next to me and he said 'see there you are, of course he didn't, of course that couldn't happen'. That's all he'd say.

The 'monsters' of media coverage are clearly present in this tale yet some details of her friend's story were at odds with the narrator's expectations about rape. In her account of a movie portrayal of rape, the narrator no longer shares her husband's simple view of rapists as monsters. The television fiction is interpreted in the light of the personal story. The divide between horrific attackers and normal men is breaking down.

Rather different is a woman who recounts how, as a teenager and heroin user on the streets of New York, she experienced an attempted rape:

This guy I went home with from a pub left the room after we'd had sex, and next thing his flatmate comes into the room naked trying to get me to sleep with him, quite forcefully, but eventually I talked him out of it, and he drove me home. I was about seventeen.

[Female, middle years]

The young woman in this tale does not meet the conventional criteria of domesticated respectability and risk avoidance that the media expect of worthy victims; rather she is asserting her rights over her own body. Yet it is also a tale characterised by its ordinariness; the assailant is talked out of rape and drives the young woman home. For this woman rapists are not monsters, they are normal men like those she now encounters in her local country town:

Respondent [female, middle years]: Well, drunk men in public bars can be pretty scary. The look in their eyes and just knowing the small mind mentality sometimes, feeling like it's a right, I get that vibes sometimes from men who have tried to pick me up and I'm not interested, their alcohol fuels their rejection or something ...
Interviewer: Do you think there's anything that can be done to make this area less dangerous?
Respondent: You could nail them to their stools by their testicles or something [laughs]. I think, maybe it's a kind of thing about

publicans and staffing, some pubs feel fine because there are people working on the door, and others are really short staffed.

In this response the focus shifts from women's sexual vulnerability to men's sexual bodies, the humour underlining the view that these are not monsters but ordinary men whose behaviour needs to be controlled. Asked about dangerous people, this respondent focuses not on unmasking the hidden rapist but on identifying a context in which alcohol tips the balance to reveal not just embodied male desire (the eyes, the testicles) but the underlying 'small-minded' beliefs that legitimise the threatened violence. She in turn counters this discourse of male rights over female bodies, not with a denial of female sexuality, but an affirmation of women's right to choose. Instead of a discourse of psychopathic monsters and risk avoidance, this respondent asserts women's rights to safety and self-determination and the community's responsibility to ensure it.

The young women that we interviewed, although varying in their preparedness to take risks, strongly asserted their right to move around safely and to be protected. Their moral frames do not encompass the code of restricted, respectable behaviour espoused by many women in Weaver *et al.*'s study. Rather some of their tales expressed outrage at the failure of authorities to protect or support young people attacked in risky situations. In a tale of rape, the risky drinking behaviour of the victim in no way justifies police indifference:

> I was talking to a friend who works with me, one of her friends had been to a party, she was a bit drunk but alright, and my friend was dancing with her, and then she went off, and they were looking for her. They went outside and they found her shivering naked in a gutter, and she'd been raped by a guy they all knew. They took her to the police station, and said, 'She's been raped, we've just found her' and he said, 'There's insubstantial evidence, but we'll charge you for underage drinking'.
>
> [Focus group, young female]

Another girl recounts police arresting her for carrying a knife on a train while ignoring a gang of males who had punched her severely in the eyes. For these young women their behaviour does not relieve the police of a duty of care and, within their own circuits of communication, outrage is expressed at authorities' indifference to young women's risk.

The young woman 'shivering naked in a gutter' is part of a pervasive discourse of female bodily vulnerability. Young women, in particular, frequently talk of their sense of vulnerability, especially when alone, as based on their smaller, weaker bodies:

> Males can be overpowering. They're bigger than females and they wouldn't really have much of a hard time holding a female down.
>
> [Young female]

Outrage as well as fear is expressed at reports of sexual assault. Rape is portrayed as posing an irreversible threat to the person which, as one young woman stated, cannot be 'cancelled like a credit card', a theme echoed by another:

> You can't buy a new body, a new soul, that why I guess it's really terrible.
>
> [Young female]

Both these young women pose and reject a discourse of commodification in favour of a discourse about ownership of one's body. An attack on the body is an attack on the person, leaving psychological scars that cannot be erased.

Extreme bodily violation (especially of a 'worthy' victim) contributes to outrage. Asked about crimes that angered them, several interviewees mentioned the much-publicised case of Anita Coby, an attractive young Sydney nurse raped and murdered while returning from work by a group of young men. One woman, struggling to explain why she favoured capital punishment in this case more certainly than for the Port Arthur killer whom she saw as psychiatrically disturbed, talked of the pleasure gained by the killers:

> But someone who goes and rapes and commits some horrific crime against somebody, really horrible with knives and things like that. It just seems to be, especially when it's of a sexual nature, in a way they're getting off on it and I just find that sick.
>
> [Female middle years]

In these tales female bodies are not just a site of risk, they are a call to action. The media themselves can be targets, not just for what they report but what remains hidden. Several groups of young women claimed that their local papers are reluctant to report the information on assault and rape in their neighbourhood that they need for their own protection, instead preferring to promote the positive community image espoused by their business clientele. Not all those demanding changes in the media's approach were younger women. An older woman talking of travelling on the trains declared:

> We give up and hide ourselves and we give the space to intruders. I think the media should reverse this attitude and tell the people to protect themselves but go ahead and not be hiding ... we should go out in masses and show body, not hide.
>
> [Focus group, older female]

Here is an alternative, bodies *en masse* as powerful not vulnerable, reclaiming public space as theirs by right:

> Let's ... say, 'This is our space, we don't want you here!'
>
> [Focus group, older female]

Both these women confront the more common voices of caution and anxiety, rejecting intimidation and asserting their right to move freely. But showing body relies on numbers, thus the almost evangelistic fervour of the few women who attempt to recruit others to a show of bodily strength.

Unworthy victims: young men at risk

The construction of the female body as a 'site of risk' has the potential for negative impact on men as well as women, obscuring the fact that not all male violence is directed at women. While women are expected to avoid risk, men are seen as strong, agentive and able to protect themselves. Several female respondents indicated a concern that their sons or partners put themselves at risk by reacting aggressively to threat, perceiving a need to defend their masculinity. Men can be further burdened by the construction of the male role as protector, several mentioning that they were more worried about crime when with a female companion. One young man cast as defender of his household and protector of his girlfriend's safety declared grave self-doubts about living up to these expectations. Men can suffer from media discourse that not only obscures their fear but minimises the trauma of violent assaults. Stanko and Hobdell (1993) have dramatically documented the impact of serious violence on male victims. The construction of the male body as strong and agentive potentially leaves male victims disempowered.

Although many of our respondents talked of their strength and physical prowess, which allowed them to move around confidently, it was not always enough. A young man, who began an account of a mugging:

> I was with two of my friends who were both big and strong and I felt really comfortable with them, they both do martial arts and stuff.

was just one of several young male respondents who told tales of threats and violent incidents particularly involving gangs of young men. A seventeen-year-old private schoolboy recounted how 'homies'[3] had invaded a party where friends had their faces smashed in and had to be hospitalised. On the previous Saturday evening, this young man and his seven mates had not been prepared to travel by train to their local station in an affluent suburb after a night out at the pub because of their fear of attack by homeboys. They instead relied on friends or parents to drive them; and our respondent called on his mother to drive him home after weekday rugby training because he didn't want to travel alone after the peak school travel period. Yet the vulnerability of these young men is obscured by their bodies; they were large six-foot rugby players, not the image of vulnerable worthy victims. The schoolboy's story was not an isolated one; many young males were involved in the strategic negotiation of public space as another young man explained:

> not to draw attention to myself in any way, not to interfere in anyone's business, not to insult anyone, not to show intimidation but not to be cocky either.
>
> [Young male]

Despite the evidence that teenagers are afraid of other teenagers, public media (as well as academic) discourses often seem polarised between a stereotype of teenagers as out of control and a desire to defend young people from this negative stereotyping. Both approaches ignore the heterogeneity among young men, which this age group itself can spot with almost anthropological precision. Thus, one nineteen-year-old male, who regularly travelled to Sydney by train to go to gigs and parties, pointed out the differences in place, dress, music and mode of address as between 'rednecks', 'westies', 'homies', 'footies'[3] and other subcultural male groups that he discussed. He knew he would meet 'rednecks' in his local pub, and that if he went there he might get into a fight over his girl. But that could be avoided simply by not going to that pub. But the 'homies' could not be avoided, because this respondent couldn't afford a car, needed to use the trains to conduct his leisure life, and 'homies' targeted the trains as a part of their own economy. He had had three incidents with 'homies' in recent months, and had adopted a specific body language and mode of address in response to their usual opening gambit of 'You looking at me?' Two out of three times this had worked for our respondent. As he described, he adopted different mundane routines according to the various socio-cultural groups that might threaten him. With the 'homies':

> You don't go out of your way to dodge people; you just keep your head down.
>
> [Young male]

It is apparent that selective and strategic use of public space is not confined to women. Many young men are also aware of risk and take 'reasonable precautions' when travelling alone at night via the kind of everyday, mundane routines in public places that Weaver *et al.* (2000) find problematic among women on the grounds that it naturalises and perpetuates their subordination. We are not claiming that young men are as constrained as young women in their everyday use of public space, but rather that the gendered portrayal of risk has implications for men as well as women. Acknowledgement that males can be fearful and can learn from women's protective strategies will impact not only on men but can empower women and challenge their subordination. Recognising threats to people, young and old, male and female, in public space can promote community responsibility for public safety rather than an individualised risk avoidance discourse. If the media is to play a role in this process, the capacity of the media for outrage needs to be harnessed.

Changing public agendas: outrage, worthy victims and a rights discourse

Understanding media coverage of crime in terms of outrage based on violation of rights (English, 1991) is not to deny that outrage can be constrained within the patriarchal assumptions surrounding risk that Weaver and her colleagues identify. Within a risk discourse only those who endeavour to minimise their risk are worthy victims, deserving of public outrage if attacked. Victims who fall short of these standards can be labelled as 'other'; they are not like us and therefore we, and our loved ones, are not at risk of their fate. Such outrage can operate within a traditional law-and-order perspective, which emphasises risk minimisation and the punishment and containment of offenders. The analysis from our fear of crime study has indicated the power but also the limitations of this construction of risk.

An alternative viewpoint adopts a rights discourse; a citizen's right to move around safely is not dependent on their personal characteristics or their risk minimisation strategies. However, any notion of outrage is embedded in a political and ideological position. The role played by outrage in challenging public policy can be explored through the varied narrative framings of an incident, referred to by several respondents, that occurred just prior to our research study. On the face of it, the shooting of an adult male carrying a knife is unlikely to provoke community outrage. Looked at more closely, a number of elements relate to Sandman's model; the death of a Frenchman shot by police on Bondi Beach was captured on video, producing a memorable and exotic location. It is the dimension of moral relevance, however, that clearly marks out this case. Only days before the incident the victim had begun to demonstrate symptoms of a psychological disorder; when hospitalised he absconded without being noticed and returned home for a knife. His friends followed him and engaged police help in an effort to protect him. Respondents in our study who talked about the incident saw the police shooting as an irresponsible overreaction and a failure of the police's duty to protect the vulnerable in the community:

> The community loses confidence in, you know, the people who are supposedly looking after us.
>
> [Older male]

In this incident the largely hidden problem of how violence by psychologically disturbed individuals is dealt with by the police was dramatically focused in a single moment of space and time. Although several respondents reacted very strongly to this incident, even labelling it a 'police crime', public debate at the time was more divided. People brought to this narrative their own experiences and attitudes; some, for example, felt outraged on behalf of the police. Moreover, many of these different moral frames were canvassed in the media. Thus, in this case, neither was the media response simple nor were the public passive absorbers of media judgements. The highly contested nature of the Frenchman's status as vulnerable victim focused a public debate about the nature of police training and strategies in response to the mentally ill.

This analysis immediately suggests a less monolithic and unidirectional view of media impact on public perceptions of crime and greater scope for challenging dominant discourses than provided by the 'strong ideological effects' approach to media power assumed in Weaver *et al.*'s essay. The strength of the concept of outrage lies in explaining why certain kinds of moral tale can generate this intense public reaction and counter-reaction. A dramatic parallel in the US was the murder of the young gay male, Matthew Shepard. His body, fighting for life, was found bound to a fence in the harsh Wyoming landscape. Anti-gay hate crimes are not unusual, yet this provoked huge media coverage generating outrage and counter-reaction: the crucifixion-like image forming a stark icon for debate about his worthy victim status. It is the combination of the distinctive elements, in Sandman's (1987b) terms, and the moral resonance of these stories that make them a focal point of public debate, the reason why some deaths provoke outrage while others only voyeuristic interest or no interest at all. Such tales can play an important role in shifting public agendas, enabling the insertion of alternative discourses into fissures and gaps in media reporting.

Equally, the discourses that have treated violence in the home as routine, privatised and 'non-systemic' and thus a personal not a community issue, have been exposed in narratives that highlight women's right to protection. The widely accepted view that women can simply leave an abusive relationship presents the 'decision' to stay as a voluntary risk. It makes such women less 'worthy' victims of violence and their assault provokes less outrage. As violence in the home becomes gradually redefined, however, as a public responsibility, women's right to safety is foregrounded and women's bodies in the private sphere are valued as worthy of protection. Narratives, sometimes re-enacted in video dramas, where fatal or near fatal consequences have resulted from inadequate police response to violence in the home, both reflect and foster public outrage and shifting public attitudes. Although our study focused on fear of crime in public space, a substantial number of respondents talked of domestic violence as one of the most prevalent of crimes. While some referred to personal experience, others indicated that the media had promoted greater public awareness and discussion of domestic violence in recent years. To attack the media as the monolithic source of women's fear of public space both relegates women to a passive role in response to media portrayals and ignores the alternative potential of media tales in promoting public outrage and diversifying circulating discourses of public debate about violence (as, for example, in many soap operas).

We began this chapter with two tales of bodies, victims of violent crime. Public outrage at the Port Arthur killings produced a climate where significant gun law reform was enacted. The Snowtown bodies created no such impact on public policy. To date the only outrage has been reserved, on the part of some community members, for a local tourist operator keen to capitalise on his town's moment in the spotlight with ghoulish souvenirs. Between the grief and outrage of Port Arthur and the fascinated indifference of Snowtown lie a range of more ambiguous stories of violence. Outrage can provoke fear, further restricting the opportunities of the more vulnerable in our society, but it can also provoke action. A body at risk is a person with rights. When tales of crime shift from an individualised discourse of risk to a social justice discourse of rights, the scope for outrage is enlarged and a wider debate about responses to crime open, up. Weaver *et al.* (2000) argue that the media creates the female body in public space as a site of risk, with the consequence that women are overconstrained and fearful in public space. Sandman's work on risk and outrage has generated communication manuals to assist companies in presenting risk to the public. Those concerned to shift public agendas about crime and public safety also need to understand ways to exploit the fissures and gaps in media coverage enabling individuals and groups in our community to gain media attention for alternative ways of looking at violence and crime in our society.

Notes

1. 'Young' indicates 16–30 years; 'middle years' indicates 30–60 years; 'older' indicates 60+ years.
2. All the quotations are taken from interviews and focus groups that were conducted as part of the Fear of Crime study (Tulloch *et al.*, 1998).
3. Groups of youths linked by different subcultural allegiances are: rednecks, political reactionaries most commonly associated with rural communities; westies, working-class youths from the western suburbs of Sydney; homies, homeboys who emerged from the American basketball cult, often ethnic Australians; footies, rugby league supporters.

References

Alasuutari, P. (ed.), (2000) *Rethinking the Media Audience*. London: Sage.

Allan, S., Adam, B. and Carter, C. (eds), (2000) *Environmental Risks and the Media*. London: Routledge.

Ang, I. (1985) *Watching Dallas: Soap Opera and the Melodramatic Imagination*. London: Methuen.

Ang, I. (1996) *Living Room Wars: Rethinking Media Audiences for a Postmodern World*. London: Routledge.

Burt, M. and Estep, R. (1981) 'Apprehension and Fear: Learning a Sense of Vulnerability'. *Sex Roles* 5: 511–22.

English, M. (1991) 'Victims, Agents and Outrage'. In J.B. Garrick and W.C. Gekler (eds) *The Analysis, Communication and Perception of Risk*. New York: Plenum Press, 199–204.

Gilchrist, E., Bannister, J., Ditton, J. and Farrall, S. (1998) 'Women and the "Fear of Crime": Challenging the Accepted Stereotype'. *British Journal of Criminology* 38: 283–98.

Kelly, L., (1996) '"It's Everywhere": Sexual Violence as a Continuum'. In S. Jackson and S. Scott (eds) *Feminism and Sexuality: A Reader*. Edinburgh: Edinburgh University Press.

Sandman, P.M. (1987a) 'Risk Communication: Facing Public Outrage' *EPA Journal* (November): 21–2.

Sandman, P.M. (1987b) 'Antipathy versus Hysteria: Public Perception of Risk'. In L.R. Batra and W. Klassen (eds) *Public Perception of Biotechnology*. Bethsada: MD Agricultural Research Institute.

Schlesinger, P., Dobash, R.E., Dobash, R.P. and Weaver, C.K. (1992) *Women Viewing Violence*. London: British Film Institute.

Stanko, E.A. (1996) 'Warnings to Women: Police Advice and Women's Safety in Britain'. *Violence Against Women* 2 (1): 5–24.

Stanko, E.A. and Hobdell, K. (1993) 'Assault on Men: Masculinity and Male Victimization'. *British Journal of Criminology* 33: 400–15.

Tulloch, J., Lupton, D., Blood, W., Tulloch, M., Jennet, C. and Enders, M. (1998) *Fear of Crime*, 2 vols. Canberra: National Campaign Against Violence and Crime Publications.

Tulloch, M. (2000) 'The Meaning of Age Differences in the Fear of Crime: Combining Quantitative and Qualitative Approaches'. *British Journal of Criminology* 40: 451–67.

Valentine, H. (1989) 'The Geography of Women's Fear'. *Area* 21, 4: 385–90.

Weaver, C.K., Carter, C. and Stanko, E. (2000) 'The Female Body at Risk: Media, Sexual Violence and the Gendering of Public Environments'. In S. Allan, B. Adam and C. Carter (eds) *Environmental Risks and the Media*. London: Routledge.

7
Ageist Ideology and Discourses of Control in Skincare Product Marketing[1]

Justine Coupland

1 Introduction: the importance of the face

The face is the part of the body most often exposed, and the part that is most often the normative focus of gaze and attention in private as well as public contexts. And the face is endowed with heavy semiotic significance; it is 'a prime symbol of the self' (Synnott, 1993: 2). Contemporary consumer culture sees much of individuals' (and particularly women's) symbolic capital as realised through their bodies (Bourdieu, 1977; Featherstone and Hepworth, 1991), and the face has an immeasurable role to play in the achievement of this capital. As Synnott puts it:

> the face is ... the principal determinant in the perception of our individual beauty or ugliness, and all that these perceptions imply for self-esteem and life-chances. (1993: 73)

My purpose here is to explore how particular aspects of the semiotic significance of bodies, and in particular faces, are shaped and influenced by the mass media. As we shall see, advertisements and features, in particular in magazines, actively impose norms and priorities for consumers' orientations to their facial and bodily appearance. Featherstone (1991) has described the media's role in imaging preferred bodily appearance as a *moral agenda*, with particular significance for the body as it ages:

> Advertising, feature articles and advice columns in magazines and newspapers ask individuals to assume responsibility for the way they look. This becomes important not just in the first flush of

adolescence and early adulthood, for notions of 'natural' bodily deterioration and the bodily betrayals that accompany ageing have become interpreted as signs of moral laxitude.

(Ibid.: 178)

As the data analysis which follows will show, individual women, in the current sociocultural climate, are consistently persuaded of two important things: one that it is undesirable to appear to be ageing; and two that they must assume responsibility to stay young-looking, or to disguise their apparent ageing. But to live in the world is to age, day by day, from birth. How can advertisers persuade women that stopping the ageing process or, rather, disguising its effects on the body is achievable?

The chapter is based on a small-scale survey of product advertisements and features in popular women's magazines, which enables me to trace several themes linked to the way in which skin care, sun-use and tanning products are marketed. A close pragmatic analysis may be able to elucidate sociocultural values for ageing and the body project (Featherstone, 1991; Giddens, 1991; Shilling, 1993). My aim is to examine the discursive means by which popular media discourses negotiate ageism as it is applied to the body, and in particular, the face. What I think emerges from the analysis is some purchase on the gendered and consumerised ways in which the semiotics of the visibly ageing face are socially constructed and reconfirmed in contemporary popular texts. My data are a corpus of high-circulation women's magazines, published in the UK between May 1999 and February 2001. Magazines were chosen for being at least partly concerned with beauty and grooming, and informally judged as aimed at a range of readership ages: *Cosmopolitan, Essentials, Family Circle, Good Housekeeping, Marie-Claire, New Woman, Prima, Red, She, Shine, Vogue* and *Zest.* I am not arguing a particular distributional case, but the texts chosen had, at the time of sampling, high prominence in the market and the issues they address continue to have media prominence at the time of writing.

The analysis will examine advertisements and features that make claims about enhancing the appearance of the body, using two main types of product. First, skincare products (mainly marketed as moisturisers) and second, sun-protection and self-tanning agents. The texts I am concerned with are clearly part of the media promotion of body culture, with the importance of bodily beauty as a taken-for-granted assumption.

Particular analytic foci will be explored as follows. In section 2, I first explore the *rhetorical voices* advertisers and feature writers use to impose and impute values and moral responsibilities on individuals' body management. Second, I turn to the question of *age-imaging* to show how such media texts cast ageing as exclusively physically realised, and as fundamentally problematic. Third, I look at rhetorical strategies linked to the *resistance of ageing* through scientised and marketised solutions. Section 3 explores the dilemma inherent in the body imperatives of tanning, the 'premature ageing' which has been associated with sun-use and the inherent dilemma this opens up for consumers in the moral imperatives of bodily self-presentation.

2 Skin care, the face and ageing

Currently, in the UK, there is a proliferation of skincare beauty products marketed specifically on the basis of claims made about controlling or reversing the effects of ageing, which both key into and reconfirm deeply entrenched sociocultural attitudes about outward signs of growing older. As we shall see, advertisements formulate the ageing process, for women at least, as some kind of correctable aberration. For example, product advertisements and features in the skincare data clearly indicate ageist assumptions in their reference to 'fine lines and wrinkles' or [loss of] 'elasticity and firmness' as problematic or errant. Lexical items like *repair* (metaphorically implicating 'broken' or 'unfit for service'), and *correction* (with its implication of error or misdemeanour) are common. These meanings are indicative of the unwatchability of old age (Woodward, 1991), as I have argued elsewhere (N. Coupland and J. Coupland, 1997a). The dominant contemporary Western response to ageing is of repression; the ageing female body is 'unwatchable', and so strategies must be found to conceal or counter the outward signs of ageing. The issue is gendered in that in contemporary Western culture women's symbolic capital is still, to a greater extent than men's, derived from their appearance. Youthful appearance is at a premium, and so visible ageing is particularly problematised for older women (Woodward, 1999). It seems to me that there are things to say about each of Texts 7.1–5 in relation to all three themes in the following discussion; rhetorical voice, age-imaging and resistance of ageing. But for the sake of clarity, I will explore these themes in turn.

2.1 Whose ideology? Rhetorical voice

In the texts that follow, ideologies about the ageing face and body are communicated at times through ambiguous authorship, which makes it unclear whose voice is 'speaking' (Goffman, 1981: 144). This ambiguity appears to be positively functional for the marketing purposes of features and advertisements, in that, irrespective of the authorial voice affected, they adopt an uncompromisingly negative stance towards ageing. This stance, as we will see, potentially reaps enormous economic benefits for the advertisers and product manufacturers (see also Coupland and Williams, 2002).

Text 7.1²
(Single-page feature. Colour visuals of young, line-free model, of the film-stars referred to on lines 13–15, and of skincare products. Extract, from *Shine*, November 1999: 27):

1   **time is on your side**
     You're approaching the end of
     your 20s- and that's great! You're
     at your gorgeous, glowing best...
5   Approaching your 30s
     is a scary time for a woman, when it
     comes to beauty. Everywhere you look
     there are images of gorgeous young
     women in their 20s looking vibrant,
10   lovely, and quite frankly, irresistible to
     men. Even though you know that there
     are plenty of sexy, gorgeous female
     role models in their 30s, think of Nicole
     Kidman and Sandra Bullock, and even
15   older, like Goldie Hawn, it's hard not to
     feel that somehow, something has
     packed up shop and gone, never to
     come back. It's true that your skin will
     never again be wrinkle-free or have
20   that same flush of youth, and you're
     probably having to work harder to feel
     fit, healthy and glowing.....

[The feature goes on to recommend three types of product for:]
'stronger, brighter hair
fresher, lighter make up
glowing skin – at any age'

Perhaps the most striking aspect of Text 7.1 is the young age at which this text constructs visible ageing as problematic. But what is the source of the rhetorical voice used to raise this 'problem'? Is it prototypical late 20s woman's 'inner' voice, scripted for her? The text certainly carries a strong ideological assumption that quite young women (twenty-some-things) are (or should be) concerned about the effects of ageing on their (in the text, *your*) appearance and desirability. The text repeatedly excludes the writer by using *you* (*everywhere you look*; *even though you know, your skin will never be ...*) (see also Fairclough, 1989 on synthetic personalisation). But although such 'you' constructions are framed as if voicing the reader's *existing* concerns and preoccupations (and therefore assuming the prescriptive voice of the reader's own conscience), the concerns these constructions express are arguably, instead, the voice of the ominiscient moral authority, as represented by the media. When the consumer reads that it is *scary* to be approaching thirty, *when it comes to beauty*, if this is not a fear already existent in the woman's inner voice, it may well be one engendered by the advertiser's authorial voice: the two become indistinguishable, a discursive strategy which seems calculated to incline the reader favourably towards aquisition of the featured products. The authorial voice in Text 7.2 is handled rather differently:

Text 7.2
(Double-page advertisement/feature; extract, from *Red* promotion, June 1999: 184/5. Lefthand page, white letters over a full-page colour face-and-shoulder photo of a very young-looking model with dreamy facial expression and smooth, translucent-looking skin):

1   When fine lines and wrinkles first start to appear, don't bypass
     the mirror in horror, move your skincare routine into the 21st
     century with Nivea Visage's revolutionary Co-Q10 range
(Facing page, whole page of text with visuals of products)
     ...ALL CHANGE PLEASE
5   If we're lucky, it isn't until our thirties that we really
     start to notice any fine lines and wrinkles. By this
     point, most of us will have been using the same
     cleanse, tone and moisturise routine for years. The
     trouble is, time has a nasty habit of catching up with
10   us in the end. But rather than spending a
     fortune on 'rejuvenating' creams that don't deliver,
     why not try caring for your skin the Nivea Visage way?

Nivea Visage has introduced a powerful active
ingredient called Co-enzyme Q10, which has previ-
15 ously been used only in medicine and as a nutritional
supplement. Generally known as Co-Q10, this miracle
molecule is naturally present in our bodies and plays
a key role in helping us convert food into energy
and combat the ageing process. Basically, a lack of
20 Co-Q10 adds up to a lot of creases and furrows
on our skin ...
... The result is a proven reduction in visible
lines and wrinkles together with improved firmness
and elasticity. Or put simply, better-looking skin.
25 So, it's true – life really does get better and better as
we get older ...

The first three lines of Text 7.2 speak with a self-evidently omniscient voice, explicitly distancing itself from the reader, with an
implied 'you' in *don't bypass the mirror* and explicit 'you'/r on lines 2
and 13. Early in the text, at lines 1–3, the voice of the moral authority is particularly clear; with the woman enjoined not to ignore *fine
lines and wrinkles* by looking away *in horror* (reminiscent of
Featherstone's idea of 'moral laxitude'?). Instead, the reader is persuaded to assume responsibility for her appearance (*move your skincare routine into the 21st century*) by purchasing so-called remediative
solutions. Then, somewhat paradoxically, after line 4, the text shifts
to a more apparently empathetic 'we' (line 5 *if we're lucky*; line 7
most of us; lines 9–10 *catching up with us in the end;* line 20–21 *creases
and furrows on our skin*) presumably in an attempt to claim a commu-
nal voice and thus disavow taking a stance of the 'moral high
ground'. But within the same text, and particularly from line 13
onward, the need to deliver a scientised message (which I will return
to in section 2.3) means adopting a voice of authority, which is
somewhat at odds with the communality, and the text therefore
takes on a somewhat hybrid style. There are, of course, other ideological aspects of Texts 7.1 and 7.2 which deserve fuller commentary, and it is to those that I now turn.

2.2   Age imaging and ageist assumptions

Texts 7.1 and 7.2, using various voices, speak to relatively young
women, in both cases to communicate ageist notions about bodily
change-over-time. In Text 7.1 *time is on your side* sends a pretty clear

message that later in life, time will be against 'you'. And, in terms of projected lifespan and its prospects, if late twenties is claimed to be *your best* the implication is that worse is to come (see lines 15ff). Text 7.1 also raises notions of inter age-group competitiveness by claiming that younger women will more easily attract mates because they are *vibrant* and *lovely* (lines 9–10). References to bodily degeneration and loss are particularly striking, even if the accompanying images are hazy: *it's hard not to feel that somehow, something has packed up shop and gone, never to come back* (lines 15–18).

Text 7.2 also reveals a strongly ageist ideology, in relation to the ageing face in particular. Although lines 1–2 do not mention the face, the later mention (line 8) of the face–skincare routine mantra *cleanse, tone and moisturise* and the name of the product (Nivea Visage) indicate that a woman will find her own ageing face unwatchable (*don't bypass the mirror in horror*). And lines 5–6 assume the desirability of delaying outward signs of ageing. From the ideological position adopted in this text, the stigmatised indices of age appear (and matter) early in the lifespan. As in Text 7.1, the twenties are implicated as the time when one of the first bodily signs of ageing are likely (unless *we're lucky*) to appear. And from this perspective, a woman must attend to (notice, and anoint) signs of ageing on her face for well over half (if not three-quarters) of her expected lifespan. In Text 7.3, ageing is pathologised, with the appearance of ageing in the face reframed as a health issue.

Text 7.3
(Double-page advertisement. Full text, from *She*, June 1999: 128/9. Lefthand page, a full-page colour photo of the face of a young, smooth-faced and line-free model with a white bandage wrapped around her face, covering her hair, temples and the edge of her cheeks, and enclosing her jawline; the words below are printed across her forehead):

1   Introducing the latest **intervention**
              in the fight against skin ageing.
Facing page, paragraph of text with visual of product:

Reti C
Pure Retinol and Pure Vitamin C.
5   **A new force in anti-ageing.**
Visible results from 15 days.

VICHY Laboratoires have perfected the first
three-phase emulsion containing Pure Retinol
and Pure Vitamin C in their stable and active forms
10   to correct the signs of ageing.

Reti C combines the rapid radiance renewal
action of Vitamin C with the wrinkle corrective
benefits of Retinol.

Use morning and/or night. Hypo-allergenic.
15   With VICHY Thermal Spa Water.
Effectiveness tested by dermatologists.

Ask your pharmacist for advice.

(offset, next to photo of product)
NEW
Patent pending

20   VICHY SOURCE OF HEALTHY SKIN

The text uses metaphors of war often associated with illness and
perhaps especially cancer (*cf.* Sontag, 1991; Gwyn, this volume) (*intervention in the fight against skin ageing,* line 1; *force in anti-ageing,* line 5).
Signs of ageing (line 10) [lack of] *radiance* (line 11) and *wrinkle*[s] (line
12) are clearly formulated as physical aberrations or errors against
which the product will provide *corrective benefits* (lines 10 and 12). The
visual of the bandage-swathed model is an image redolent of sterile
treatment at the hands of trained medical experts, and the last two
lines (16 and 17) of the main text read: *Effectiveness tested by dermatologists; Ask your pharmacist for advice.* The first of these evokes medically
trained skin experts and the second is an imprecation more usually
associated with health issues. Readers are likely to confer more expertise and objectivity on the pharmacist than the beautician. It is
difficult not to conclude that the look of ageing (if not ageing itself) is
being pathologised here, with the (quite naturally) ageing body being
reconstrued as the (preventably) ailing body, in need of the available
pharmaceutical intervention.

Until relatively recently, 'anti-ageing' skin care marketing has
focused almost entirely on the face and (to a lesser extent) the hands.[3]
Text 7.4 refers first to the *body*; (used, as it seems from the visual, to
refer to the torso and limbs); second to the *hands*, and third to the *lips.*)
In this text, the advertisers enumerate (and, in due course, with the aid

of the products, claim to obliterate) seven outward signs of bodily ageing, in a continuation of an earlier advertising campaign (directed at the ageing face) by the same company.

Text 7.4
(A twelve-page pamphlet, stapled into the magazine. Extract, from *New Woman*, February 2001. On the cover: white capitals on a plain black background):

1   YOU'VE DISCOVERED HOW TO
          REDUCE THE APPEARANCE OF
     SEVEN SIGNS OF AGEING
               ON YOUR FACE
5   **NOW** IT'S TIME TO DISCOVER ... OIL OF OLAY

(First page, with visuals: three young-looking models, one in a brief silk slip displaying her limbs, one lifting her hands to her face, and one whose lips are darkly and prominently painted.)
     ... HOW TO **REDUCE**
          THE APPEARANCE OF
          SEVEN SIGNS OF AGEING
     ON YOUR **BODY**, ON YOUR **HANDS**
10   AND ON YOUR **LIPS**
(Next page, with visual of product)
11   TOTAL EFFECTS BODY **ANTI-AGEING MOISTURISING TREATMENT**
     Because skin ageing doesn't begin and end on the face, **total effects
     body treatment** tackles the appearance of ageing, especially on areas
     you need it most, such as the **chest, elbows, knees, and heels**.
15   *'Works the same magic as the moisturiser'*
                                                        ELLE recommends
     NEW TOTAL EFFECTS BODY TREATMENT WITH VITANIACIN
     • INTENSIVELY HYDRATES DRY SKIN
     • IMPROVES SKIN'S FIRMNESS
20   • VISIBLY REDUCES THE APPEARANCE OF FINE LINES AND WRINKLES
     • VISIBLY EVENS SKIN TONE
     • HELPS DIMINISH THE APPEARANCE OF BLOTCHES AND AGE SPOTS
     • SOFTENS AND SMOOTHES SKIN TEXTURE
     • TRANSFORMS SKIN DULLNESS TO A MORE YOUTHFUL HEALTHY
       GLOW
25   PROVEN TO REDUCE THE APPEARANCE OF 7 SIGNS OF AGEING
(opposite page, visual of young-looking model in brief silk slip)
     TOTAL EFFECTS
     IT'S ALL OVER
     FOR **SEVEN SIGNS**
29   OF **BODY** AGEING

(The pamphlet also gives similar coverage of 'hand treatment' ('To tell a woman's age, they used to say, look at her hands') and 'full treatment lipcolour' ('The seven signs of ageing don't stop at your lip line. Lips are ageing too'). Each product is promised as PROVEN TO REDUCE THE APPEARANCE OF THE 7 SIGNS OF AGEING).

Text 7.4 is explicitly anti-ageing (line 11). And the specificity and repetition of the catch-phrase *seven signs of ageing* insistently reifies this category system. In Text 7.4, the ageing face is acknowledged as of primary importance as an issue of concern, but for the moment backgrounded (line 4), with other parts of the body foregrounded as signifiers of apparent ageing: *skin ageing doesn't begin and end on the face* (line 12). The battle metaphor (*cf.* Text 7.2) is again used for the relationship between the woman's body and the product (line 13, *tackles*). And arguably, again we see indications of the moral imperative (*you need it*, line 13) to control signs of ageing in: *tackles the appearance of ageing, especially on areas you need it most, such as the chest, elbows, knees, and heels* (lines 13–14).

But the reified *seven signs of ageing* must be inferred by the reader from the list of seven benefits of the product (lines 18–24). In the order of the list, these would comprise: dry skin; lack of muscle tone (firmness); fine lines and wrinkles; uneven skin tone; blotches and age spots;[4] rough or hard skin texture; and dull skin. Those which are not conventionally or stereotypically associated with bodily ageing (and do not tend to appear in other adverts) are *dry skin, uneven skin tone* and *rough skin*. It seems that only the bodies of the youngest of babies will not have these last three. This observation might lead us to ask just how young women's skin must look in order to escape the stigma of signs of bodily ageing, and to suggest that the imperatives here are hopelessly unattainable.

Ageism is prominent in a far wider range of features and advertisements on skincare products than space allows me to examine in detail. As Texts 7.1–4 have indicated, first, the ageing body is pathologised. Secondly, the appearance of ageing is equated with ageing itself, as if the effects of time and living on the observable body (or the body that is the object of gaze) are the only significant elements or experiences of ageing. And thirdly, consumers are assumed to find their own ageing unwatchable. The texts we have examined so far have already begun to show how 'solutions' to these 'problems' are preferred.

2.3 Resistance of ageing: marketing scientised 'solutions'

In Text 7.1, we saw that references to the passing look of youth (*flush*) and signs of ageing (*wrinkles*) are allied to the notion of bodily *work and responsibility* (*you're probably having to work harder*, line 21). In the data collected, features and advertisements work to persuade women readers that they must take responsibility for controlling or reversing the bodily signs of ageing, specifically by using skincare beauty products marketed on that basis. A significant part of how this is achieved is by advertisers claiming authenticity and marketability for their products through foregrounding the scientific or clinical aspects of product manufacture and testing, as in Texts 7.2, 3 and 5.

In these texts, the marketised solution is scientised (Chaiken, 1987). For example, in Text 7.2, line 3 the product is said to contain *a powerful active ingredient called Co-enzyme 10*) (and see also lines 13ff). It is claimed that this product is derived from the realms (the laboratories, perhaps) of medicine and food science (lines 15–16). From lines 16ff, the text continues to draw on a scientised register to persuade the potential consumer that she is being offered access to a *miracle molecule* (17–18) (though note here the conflation of science and magic). In addition, the science is allied to the notion of a 'natural' element (*naturally present in our bodies*, line 17) to *combat the ageing process* (line 19). Arguably, the implication here is that the product will be safe to use as the user will only be augmenting what her body is already doing, but with less efficiency or success than when she was younger (lines 18–20) (see also Coupland and Williams, 2002). Later, too, the text draws from a register of objective, experimental science: *result*; *proven* (lines 23–24). In all, the text tells us that the look of ageing is degenerative, and so the ageing body needs scientifically researched, marketised help to *combat the ageing process* (line 19) and give the consumer *better-looking skin* (line 24); for 'better-looking' read 'younger-looking'. This adds up to the assumption made in the final sentence: as women grow older, an improved quality of life is dependent on staving off the signs of ageing.

Even more than Text 7.2, Text 7.3 is heavily scientised, framed by reference to registers of medicine and pharmacy. The technical-sounding product references emerge from lines 7ff.: *three-phase emulsion; Pure Retinol and Pure Vitamin C in their stable and active forms; Patent pending*. It seems unlikely that the average lay reader will fully understand the terms being used here. Undoubtedly the specialised terminology is designed to communicate competence and expertise, and promote confidence in Retinol and Vitamin C as 'age-correcting' agents.

However, there is a paradox surrounding the claims made in such skincare advertisements. Manufacturers are strategising in a fiercely competitive and potentially highly profitable market; even while, in the popular press and elsewhere, dermatologists and other interested parties are expressing concern that claims made in such product marketing are at best exaggerated and at worst unfounded. Germaine Greer, in her feminist polemic *The Whole Woman* (1999: 28–9), goes so far as to say:

> Women are exhorted to fight and deny their age by every means in their power. Consumer research regularly reports that nothing applied to the surface of the skin can affect the underlying structures or prevent ageing, and still the anti-ageing products continue to sell ... It must be a sad world when what every mother wants for mother's day is a 'younger-looking skin'.
> [A reference to a television advertisement for Oil of Olay moisturiser which was showing at the time Greer's book was written] That is one thing she is never going to have, even if she endures the agonies of a face lift.

And, to give another example, from an article entitled 'Holding Back the Years' journalist Richard Girling (1999) cites a consultant dermatologist:

> Anti-ageing creams? No, they don't work. By their nature cosmetics are ephemeral. What's the evidence that rubbing vitamin A on the skin has any effect? That's all retinol is, but of course people wouldn't buy it if it was just called vitamin A. That's the marketing boys for you.

The cover of the relevant *Sunday Times* supplement shows a head-and-shoulders colour photograph of a woman, her head covered with a brown paper bag, a letterbox shaped hole torn in the bag as an eyehole, and the caption:

> FACE FACTS! You want to stop skin ageing? Spend £300 on the latest cream. Now throw it away and use the bag it came in.[5]

Despite this, the discourse of anti-ageing skincare advertisements continues to make confident claims for efficacy characteristically borrowing from medical and/or pharmaceutical registers. The legalistic strategy is to mitigate these claims using carefully designed attenuating markers, as Texts 7.4 and 7.5 show.

Text 7.5

(Double-page advertisement. Full text, from *Vogue* May 1999:4/5. Lefthand page, a full-page black-and-white photo of the face of smiling, carefree-looking, line-free Elizabeth Hurley; no text.

Facing page; large colour photo of product, multiple bottles, progressively disappearing to white; half page of text beneath):

1   Now see lines and wrinkles
                   visibly reduced by up to 50%.

Diminish
Anti-Wrinkle Retinol* Treatment

5   Use Diminish nightly and the unique 3 vitamin formula time
releases Retinol into the skin minimising wrinkles visibly –
without irritation. After 8 weeks, tests show 50% reduction in
appearance of fine lines and wrinkles. Age spots seem to fade.

    *Retinol, the purest form of Vitamin A, is one of the most effec-
10 tive ingredients to reduce the visible signs of ageing.

ESTÉE LAUDER

In Text 7.5, specific lexical attenuators offset the empirically based claims: *visibly* (lines 2 and 6) in *now see lines and wrinkles visibly reduced by up to 50%* (lines 1–2); *seem* (line 8) in *age spots seem to fade; appearance* (line 8) in *50% reduction in the appearance of fine lines*. But this is carefully managed; the consumer is led to believe she will obtain control over her ageing appearance with this product, by the name of the product itself, *Diminish*, coupled with the strongly empiricist framing *After 8 weeks, tests show 50% reduction in the appearance of fine lines and wrinkles*. The mitigatory elements *visibly*, *seem* and *appearance* are echoed in Text 7.4, where *visibly* and (repeatedly, *appearance*) are also used. Presumably advertisers are claiming that it is the *look* of a face that changes, while appearing to claim that the face *itself* changes. This opens up the question of *real* versus *apparent* aspects of appearance. Text 7.5 appears to tell the consumer that applying the 'treatment' to the face inevitably occasions a local temporary change. Yet this is perplexing in the context of the 'evidence' presented on the time-cumulative effects of the product: *After 8 weeks, tests show 50% reduction in the appearance of fine lines.* Discourses of control in products marketed to reduce skin ageing are unlikely to be able to sustain coherence, we might conclude. But there are more fundamental contradictions in skincare product marketing, as we shall see in the following section.

3   Tanning

3.1   Incompatibilities: skincare, sun-use and the appearance of ageing

The texts we have examined so far work to equate beauty and desirability with youthful-looking (smooth, firm, wrinkle and blemish-free) skin on the face and body. But another set of ideologically linked features and advertisements address the equation of beauty and desirability with bodily colouration, or the acquisition of tanned skin through sun-use. Text 7.6 exemplifies the dilemma inherent within these two body project imperatives (N. Coupland and J. Coupland, 1997b), where skin ageing is largely equated with sun damage, but again with marketised solutions:

Text 7.6
(Single-page advertisement. A large colour photograph shows a line-free model, perhaps in her thirties, holding a smaller black-and-white photo, apparently of her younger self, in this photo laughing while sunbathing on a beach.
Full text from *Red*, June 1999: 179):

1   It took years to understand sun ageing.
    It takes 8 weeks to correct the signs.

    Years ago, nobody knew
    the extent to which the sun
5   caused skin ageing.
    Now, thanks to its exclu-
    sive Retinol and multi-
    vitamin formula, Neutrogena
    UV Ageing Repair Treatment
10 visibly reduces the signs of
    this sun damage. In 8 weeks,

the appearance of wrinkles,
fine lines and age spots is
reduced. Leaving your skin
15 looking firmer, younger and
healthier.

(Visual of product; showing following text)

NEW Neutrogena
UV AGEING
REPAIR
20 TREATMENT
RETINOL AND MULTI-VITAMIN
DERMATOLOGICAL
FORMULA

Neutrogena
25 Recommended by dermatologists

Text 7.6 is in no doubt that sun-use ages the skin, *cf. sun ageing* (line 1) and *the extent to which the sun caused skin ageing* (lines 4–5). In (line 11) *this sun damage* is by implication described as *wrinkles, fine lines and age spots* (lines 12–13). As in other skincare adverts, we see metaphors of skin ageing as error or broken-ness: *correct* (line 2) *Repair* (line 9 and 19) and indications of clinical involvement in *Treatment* (line 20) and *Dermatological Formula* (lines 22–3). In addition, the reference to *healthier-*looking skin (line 16) suggests that older-looking skin is less healthy-looking, equating youthfulness not just with beauty but also with health.

In our earlier essay (N. Coupland and J. Coupland, 1997b) we considered sun-use in the context of bodily risk factors, 'premature' ageing and melanoma. But despite widespread knowledge (as referred to in Text 7.6) about prolonged exposure to the sun causing 'premature ageing', and even despite well-publicised health dangers about skin cancer, large numbers of current advertisements and features in women's magazines (particularly during the summer months) tend to restate the proposition that a tanned body is a beautiful and desirable body, and even a healthy body. Consumerised discourses are, then, currently actively encouraging two conflicting body projects. First, the long-term body project of maintaining youthful-looking skin (skin which is undamaged by the sun), and second, the short-term body project of acquiring tanned skin. The economic potential of marketing products and ideas that promote skin damage *and* products and ideas that rectify skin damage are obvious. Over the last few years, as an antidote to the ultimately damaging goal of tanning, there has been some evidence in popular media texts of revision of self-presentational ideals, specifically in redefining the desirability of fair skin. This has gained some credence, partly through media accolades of well-known film-stars and models (such as Nicole Kidman and Sophie Dahl) for their 'alabaster skin', but, overall, tanned skin still appears to hold greater sway in the body marketplace.[6]

Consumers have no reason to relinquish tanning goals if they are offered persuasive evidence that they can purchase ways to allow them to tan without damaging their skin. A *Zest* feature (June 1999: 28–32) 'Colour Blind? Why the Safe Sun Message Still Hasn't Sunk In' claims (under the heading '4 things you may not know about sunbathing') that the sun 'causes 90% of visible ageing ... the skin starts to sag and wrinkles start to develop'. But despite categorically linking 'prematurely' ageing skin to sun-use, later the *Zest* feature promotes marketised 'solutions' to the dilemma in the shape of sunscreening agents: 'Torn between looking tanned and ensuring the health of your skin? Here's how you can do both.' Clearly, features and advertisements are still proclaiming the feasibility of 'safe tanning' over a decade after the risks of melanoma and skin ageing first became widely known. The non-sequitur, as it must be, of pursuing the long-term body project of maintaining youthful-looking skin, while still rejecting the desirability of fair skin, is expressed in the following extract:

Text 7.7

(Single-page advert/promotion; extract, from *Zest: The Health and Beauty Magazine* June 1999 p 121. On righthand side of page, colour photo of tanned, young model sunbathing in swimming costume on beach):

1   White may be a fashion favourite but as far as beauty and
     the colour of our skin is concerned, most of us still prefer more of
     a sexy golden tone. But how do we achieve it while protecting our
     precious skin from the damaging effects of the sun? Boots Soltan
5   has the solution with a relaunched, reformulated range of suncare
     products that not only offer ultimate protection and a wonderful
     tan but are convenient to use and feel fabulous at the same time...
     Protecting
     For a start, Boots Soltan products give excellent
10   protection against both the burning UVB rays and
     the damaging UVA rays that penetrate deep into
     the skin causing premature ageing and wrinkles.

The range also contains a new Cell Protection
System with an anti-free radical agent that helps
15   to protect your skin deep down, boosting its own
natural defence system. In other words, it actually
helps your skin to defend itself ...

Tan-coloured skin (here described as a *golden tone*, line 3) is ostensibly preferred, by *most of us* (line 2) to *white* skin (line 1). Here, having a tan is linked not just with *beauty* (line 1) but with looking *sexy* (line 3). The importance attached to skin protection is clear *in our precious skin* (lines 3–4), and associated risk factors are acknowledged in *damaging effects of the sun* (line 4) but marketised solutions to the dilemma unproblematically claim protection against *premature ageing and wrinkles* (line 12). The importance of the body here is paramount. Text 7.7 casts the body as precious, as a source of gratification, as a sex device, with science cast as saviour in aiding the body's natural self-protective properties.

The promotion of the suncare product in Text 7.7, as in countless other adverts, revolves around the notion of *protection*, as in the promise of *ultimate protection and a wonderful tan* (line 6–7). But the products depicted in Text 7.7 offer only very low sun protection, at factor 8 and factor 15, given that sun screens with protection factors as high as 60 are quite widely available (and agents with factors higher than 30 are sometimes misleadingly marketed as sun 'blocks'). And there is some evidence to show quite widespread public awareness that the only 'ultimate protection' from sun damage is to cover up or stay out of the sun, even though awareness often does not lead to compliance (J. Coupland, *et al.* 1998). The dilemma is clear, but what other solutions can the female body turn to?

3.2   New approaches: faking it, naturally

Apart from sun 'protection' or screening products, the alternative consumerised solution to the dilemma of wanting tanned skin (the short-term body project) and wanting skin that is undamaged by the sun (the long-term body project) is offered by products that simulate the sun's colouration of the skin. Over the last few years, and in the context of the vogue for 'naturalness', these products have resolutely avoided marketing themselves as 'fake tans'. They have instead been marketed as 'self-tanning' or 'self-action tanning' products (J. Coupland and N. Coupland, 2000). Text 7.8 promotes products by the same cosmetics company, and using the same model as Text 7.5, with the body-project aims of these two arguably complementary: the consumer (like the model) who uses both products can theoretically acquire a tan even while repairing existing sun damage *and* avoiding 'new' damage. Incidentally, the light colour of the tan depicted on Hurley's body in Text 7.8 may well be indicative of recent fashion preferences about skin colour change.[7]

Text 7.8

(Double-page advertisement. Text from *Good Housekeeping* June 1999: 4–5. Lefthand page, a full-page colour photo of a smiling Elizabeth Hurley, lightly tanned and wearing a white bathing costume sitting on a white settee; no text):

(Facing page, visuals of products and a paragraph of text)

1   Improved colour. Proven protection.*
     Self-Action SuperTan
     New from Estée Lauder Research

       Now there's a unique new idea: double-action self-tanning. With this
5   exclusive Estée Lauder formula, your skin develops rich, golden colour
       that also acts to help screen out daily exposure to UVA rays, a primary
       cause of visible skin-ageing.

       *An independent study at a world-famous university has proven that the
       advanced technology in Self-Action SuperTan helps prevent UVA damage
10   Does not replace your regular SPF sun protection.

                    ESTÉE LAUDER

Text 7.8 ostensibly offers a high level of control to the consumer. The *unique new idea* referred to in line 4 is the *double-action* the product undertakes to effect; first, by changing the user's skin colour to tan: *your skin develops rich, golden colour* and second, by affording protection from the sun. However, although heavily scientised (see especially the asterisked 'footnote') the claims made about protection are in strongly mitigated form: *acts to help screen out ... UVA rays* (line 6; see also lines 9–10). Given that the footnote seems to indicate that the usual sun-protection products are needed, it is the tanning agent that achieves prominence here, initially with the opening words *Improved colour*. This is most likely an attempt to differentiate the product from earlier 'fake' tans which were heavily stigmatised for not imitating a 'real' (sun-acquired) tan accurately enough, an issue which appears to retain some importance in the body marketplace. Even though, in the context of known risk, a tan may be seen as politically incorrect, beauty and fashion imperatives dictate a rejection of pale skin. In addition, a 'fake' or 'self-tan' must look like a real or sun-acquired tan in order to achieve culturally approved bodily appearance for the user. So the consumer is persuaded to purchase at least two products in pursuit of these complicated body goals; a new one to colour her skin and to 'help screen', even while she is warned that she must continue to purchase her 'regular sun protection' or she may unwittingly acquire a real tan and the skin damage that brings with it.

And yet the acquisition of a 'real' tan is to some extent a class issue, in the British context at least (N. Coupland and J. Coupland, 1997b: 17). The tan did not acquire fashionable desirability until around fifty years ago, when Hollywood made tanned skin fashionable through its association with leisure, hedonism and glamour. Until that time, the middle class (and particularly 'ladies') were marked off from the labouring classes by the valued paleness of their skin. Recent discourses of risk to some extent indicate that there is a return to that class distinction, with tanned bodies (especially deep tans) indicating political incorrectness, and being rejected by some upper-middle-class women and magazines aimed at them. There is, for example, a flavour of this in a recent *Vogue* feature, which foregrounds body priorities and the issue of control:

Text 7.9
(Single-page feature; extract from *Vogue*, May 1999: 87.
On lefthand side of page is the text. On righthand side of page, a large colour photograph. At bottom of page, a trio of small colour photos. All are of the faces of young catwalk models [designers' names are captioned below each] and all are tanned):

1   **VOGUE**
     beauty
     THE FAKE'S PROGRESS

     Real tans are taboo. If you want to be brown this
5   summer, make sure you're faking it. By Kathy Phillips.

     Who would have thought that a George Hamilton
     tan would be the inspiration of the season? There's
     no doubt that the crème brulée-coloured skin tone
     – which made the models on the catwalk look like
10   they'd just stepped off a Santa Monica beach –
     was as directional as any of the beaded denims
     and peasant skirts seen at the spring/summer

shows. (Not that *Vogue* is advocating a stint in
the sun – we all know that's off limits.)
15 Backstage, the make-up mavens were busy
faking it *par excellence*.........
[product recommendations follow].....
.... By the time each girl
stepped onto the runway, her wind-
blown holiday image was as expertly
20 faked as Pamela Anderson's cleavage.
We love you, George.

In the discursive position argued in Text 7.9, we see an ideology that is
obsessed with bodily appearance but responds principally to risk, and
thus categorically rejects sun-use (*Real tans are taboo* line 4, *a stint in the
sun – we all know that's off limits*, lines 13–14). The text is making its
argument from a context that has earlier assumed that fair skin was
(both politically and fashionwise) the appropriate bodily display. But
in this instance, a tan re-emerges from its status as a self-presentational
misdemeanour (as, it seems *Vogue* has previously cast it) to be reframed
as a seasonal fashion item (*directional*, line 11); a bodily adornment as
easily acquired and cast aside as a must-have item of new clothing,
make-up or temporary hair colour. Even the mode of description of the
tan colour is reminiscent of the fashion stylist (skin that looks good
enough to drool over, perhaps? *the crème brulée-coloured skin tone*, line
8). But next season, or next year, the appearance of a tan could be 'out'
again (*the inspiration of the season*, line 7). The seasonal theme is echoed
and underlined by the evocation of summer hedonism and leisure: *like
they'd just stepped off a Santa Monica beach* (line 10) and *holiday image*
(line 19), and the link with Hollywood is established with a somewhat
ironic reference to George Hamilton, an actor notorious for his year-
round deep mahogany-coloured tan.

This ideological stance allows the reappropriation of the lexical item
'fake' in 'fake' tan. Now the term becomes an index of political correct-
ness, similar in function to 'fake fur', in that each of the following
instances of fake is collocated with positive next-items: (*make sure
you're faking it*, line 5, *faking it*, par excellence, line 16, *expertly faked*,
lines 19–20). There is indeed some evidence that 'faking' is also re-
emerging in product advertisements, e.g., a Laboratoires Garnier 1999
Ambre Solaire advertisement shows a pair of heavily tanned woman's
legs with the slogan 'No one will ever know you're faking it.' But in
terms of body politics there is something of a dilemma here, too, in

that fake tan users in this realm of discourse may well want others to know their tan is a 'politically correct' or 'long-term' body-project tan.

4 Conclusion

In the texts we have considered, the body, mainly but not exclusively the face, emerges as a locus for a range of interconnected ideological practices, with features and advertisements expressing ideological positions along several dimensions. The texts have shown us that in the relationship between woman, the body and skincare products there are always issues of control, agency or responsibility involved. The advertisements and features speak from authoritative positions, though variably: at times framed as if speaking with the voice of the individual conscience, at times the voice of the female consensus, at times with the omniscient voice of authority, which refers to moral imperatives, and itself makes use of the voice of scientific expertise.

Then, the body and the face are constructed to have special significance in the prospect of ageing. The face (significantly more than other bodily parts) is treated as an age signifier, which needs work to resist the disease or enemy of ageing. Consumers can buy the means of managing their faces. In this guise, marketised versions of science enable women to do physicalised display, oriented to beauty, a sexy, healthy appearance, and always to preserve or feign the appearance of youthfulness. It is not, of course, difficult to see the self-serving cycle for the advertisers in all this.

But beyond that, and in the different domains of anti-ageing and tanning products, it is obvious that face/age ideologies throw up internal conflicts. From this point of view, the texts are most interesting for their unsubtle attempts to paper over the ideological cracks. Promoting *and* remediating skin problems cannot ultimately find a discourse to sustain it, and needs to use particular rhetorical devices to deflect litigation.

Thus, gendered bodily imperatives cause dilemmas over fulfilling short-term versus long-term body projects, and wield a kind of tyranny even over women as young as twenty.[8] Women (in particular women) have to come to terms on a personal level with how to resolve the conflicting bodily imperatives that so dominate contemporary cultural priorities, beliefs and behaviours (including, of course, shopping behaviours; Greer, 1999). To challenge these imperatives would involve a real cultural shift and present real challenges to our cognitive and conceptual frameworks (see also Hepworth, this volume). This would most obviously involve a move away from seeing the visibly ageing body as a signifier of a failing or an insignificant self, and towards embracing other models for living later life that leave us feeling comfortable with and in our changing faces and bodies.

Notes

1. Thanks are due to Nik Coupland and Peter Garrett for comments on an earlier version of this chapter.
2. The orthography and layout of advertisements and features are reproduced as closely as possible to the originals, including line breaks, bold and capital type-face etc. 'Extract' indicates that only part of the feature/advertisement is reproduced; 'Full text' indicates that the whole feature/advertisement is reproduced. Vertical dots show where text has been omitted.
3. A recent advertisement for hand cream shares many features with advertisements for products designed to be used on the face. *New Hands UV Ageing Repair Hand Treatment Visibly reduces and helps prevent the signs of ageing on hands ... with pro-retinol, AHA and multivitamins, that helps reduce the appearance of fine lines and brown spots (Good Housekeeping,* February 2001).
4. 'Age spots' seems to be a uniquely specific lexical item for the ageing appearance of bodily features. I have never seen wrinkles referred to as 'age lines' or loose skin underneath the eyes as 'age bags'. A widely heard informal term for older people is, however, 'wrinklies', pejorative in that it categorises people by one of their appearance features, reminiscent of insults yelled in the school playground.
5. Richard Girling in the *Sunday Times* (25 April 1999: 23) writes: 'Where marketing hype collides with the language of science, a new argot emerges that is the equivalent of a conjurer's mirror: it can make you see meanings that aren't really there. The Advertising Standards Authority (ASA) allows 'supportable' claims that cosmetics can have an effect on skin changes caused by 'environmental factors' (namely, sun damage); that they can temporarily prevent, delay or mask premature ageing; and that moisturisers can reduce the appearance of fine lines and wrinkles. The key words here are:
   Environmental – it is not permissible to suggest that a product can affect natural or 'intrinsic' ageing;
   Temporarily – advertisers may not claim that their products will cause permanent change;
   Prevent – they must not suggest that a product can 'reverse' environmental ageing;
   Reduce and *appearance* – they must not suggest a therapeutic effect that could actually cause wrinkles to disappear (anything that could do that would, by definition, be a medicine).'
6. 'We're probably still a long way from a time when milky, pale skin will be sexy and sought after, but at least the message is slowly but surely getting through' (Christopher New, Skin Cancer Manager for the Health Education Authority, *Zest,* June 1999: 29).
7. 'Although we still associate a tan with sex appeal, the type of tan we aspire to has changed. Gone are the days of ultra-deep tans, they're just no longer

fashionable. Instead a light, golden glow is perceived as attractive and fake tans are increasingly popular' (Debbie Then, US social psychologist, *Zest,* June 1999: 29).

8. During a small-scale pilot interview survey, a female informant, when asked about her reaction to skincare advertisements focused on ageing, responded quite vociferously: 'It's irritating when they [go] on about younger-looking skin. Why can't you have skin that looks the same age as you are? Men don't worry about having younger-looking skin. Why do I have to beat myself up if I look 37 instead of 27?'

References

Bourdieu, P. (1977) *Outline of a Theory of Practice.* Cambridge: Cambridge University Press.

Bytheway, B. and Johnson, J. (1998) 'The Sight of Age'. In S. Nettleton and J. Watson (eds) *The Body in Everyday Life.* Routledge: London.

Chaiken, S. (1987) 'The Heuristic Model of Persuasion'. In M.P. Zanna, J.M. Olson and C.P. Herman (eds) *Social Influence: The Ontario Symposium,* vol. 5, 3–40. Hillsdale, NJ: Erlbaum.

Coupland, J., Holmes, J. and Coupland, N. (1998) 'Negotiating Sun Use: Constructing Consistency and Managing Inconsistency'. *Journal of Pragmatics* 30: 699–721.

Coupland, J. and Coupland, N. (2000) 'Selling Control: Ideological Dilemmas of Sun Tanning, Risk and Leisure'. In S. Allan, C. Carter and B. Adam (eds) *Environmental Risks and the Media.* London: Routledge, 145–59.

Coupland, J. and Williams, A. (2002) 'Conflicting Discourses, Shifting Ideologies: Pharmaceutical, "Alternative" and Emancipatory Texts on the Menopause'. *Discourse and Society* 13, 4 419–446.

Coupland, N. and Coupland, J. (1997a) 'Discourses of the Unsayable: Death Implicative Talk in Geriatric Medical Consultations'. In A. Jaworski (ed.) *Silence: Interdisciplinary Perspectives.* Berlin: Mouton de Gruyter, 117–52.

Coupland, N. and Coupland, J. (1997b) 'Bodies, Beaches and Burn Times: "Environmentalism" and its Discursive Competitors'. *Discourse and Society* 8(1): 7–25.

Fairclough, N. (1989) *Language and Power.* London: Longman.

Featherstone, M. (1991) 'The Body in Consumer Culture'. In M. Featherstone, M. Hepworth and B. Turner (eds) *The Body: Social Process and Cultural Theory,* pp. 170–96.

Featherstone, M. and Hepworth, M. (1991) 'The Mask of Ageing and the Postmodern Life Course'. In M. Featherstone, M. Hepworth and B. Turner (eds.) *The Body: Social Process and Cultural Theory,* 371–89.

Giddens, A. (1991) *Modernity and Self-identity: Self and Society in the Late Modern Age.* Cambridge: Polity Press.

Girling, R. (1999) 'Holding Back the Years'. *Sunday Times,* 25 April, 18–23.

Goffman, E. (1981) *Forms of Talk.* Oxford: Basil Blackwell.

Greer, G. (1999) *The Whole Woman.* London: Anchor.

Shilling, C. (1993) *The Body and Social Theory.* London: Sage.

Sontag, S. (1991) *Illness as Metaphor/AIDS and its Metaphors.* Harmondsworth: Penguin.

Synnott, A. (1993) *The Body Social: Symbolism, Self and Society.* London: Routledge.

Woodward, K. (1991) *Aging and its Discontents: Freud and Other Fictions.* Bloomington, IN: Indiana University Press.

Woodward, K. (1999) *Figuring Age: Women, Bodies, Generations.* Bloomington, IN: Indiana University Press.

8
Talking Bodies: Invoking the Ideal in the BBC *Naked* Programme

Adam Jaworski

Introduction

The BBC series *Naked*, produced and directed by Lucy Blakstad, shown in the UK on BBC2 in November and December 1998, consists of four parts: 'Eighteen 'till I Die'; 'Prime of Your Life'; 'Hormones Going Haywire'; and 'Sod the Wrinkles'. It is a collage of interviews about people's own bodies. The fact that *Naked* consists of four parts focusing, roughly, on four different age-groups: the middle-aged; young adults; teenagers; and the elderly, appears to be the director's meta-commentary on the salience of age in all the interviews, as will become apparent in the extracts below.

The interviewees were recruited through advertisements placed in *Time Out* magazine, gyms and social clubs. About 500 individuals were interviewed, with about thirty of the 'most interesting' making it to the final version of each segment (Edwards, 1998; Midgley, 1998). Some extracts from interviews are only five to ten seconds long, while others last up to several minutes. Sometimes, the interviewees speak on camera (usually with their clothes on). Sometimes, they talk off-camera and the viewer is exposed to the images of the interviewee's naked body, usually in close up, the camera moving slowly, focusing on different parts of the body.

The programme allows us to gain an insight into a wide range of issues concerning 'discourses of the body' in a late modern, post-industrial society (namely, the UK). Although it must be remembered that the participating individuals constitute a self-selected group, who need not be representative of the society at large, the intention of the author of the programme was to make it appealing to a mass audience by striking a chord with the viewers' perceptions of their own bodies:

Blakstad ... says that Naked is about 'anxieties, obsessions, hang-ups, loves, hates, everything you feel about your body. I'm hoping that when people watch this series, they will see something of themselves, and rush to the mirror and have a look at their naked bodies'.

(Joseph, 1998: 55)

One of the means through which Blakstad probably succeeds in meeting her objectives is by interviewing 'ordinary' people. The discursive representations of the body in the *Naked* programme are 'lay' rather than 'expert' or 'scientific'. This is not to say that they are not informed by the scientific, medical and other forms of public (especially commercial: see Coupland, this volume) discourses of the body. And, as has been argued by Foucault (1978; 1979), body representations, both lay and scientific, are guided by similar truth-seeking principles leading to modes of regulation, containment, incitement and resistance. As such, these representations turn bodies from purely *natural* to socially *constructed* entities (Lupton, 2000), constrained by relations of power (Foucault's systems of knowledge or knowledge production) and by social and material inequality (see Urla and Terry, 1995: 3).

The reflexivity of *Naked* is consistent with other forms of reflexivity associated with the late-modern era (Giddens, 1990, 1991; Beck, 1992, 1994). The speaking subjects' reflexivity allows them to tackle their anxieties and uncertainties of the changing beliefs, value systems and their own shifting identities as seen and experienced through their bodies (Lupton and Tulloch, 1998).

'Normal' and 'deviant' bodies

The starting point for this chapter is the assumption drawn from Urla and Terry (1995) on the non-essentialist distinction that they make between 'normal' and 'deviant' bodies. The power constraints imposed on body representations have led to the widespread acceptance of a binary split between acceptable and unacceptable body images: 'normal' *vs.* 'deviant', or 'healthy' *vs.* 'pathological'. Such dichotomous orthodoxy has ultimately lead to the biological, anthropometric or 'bodily' explanations for 'moral deficiencies and deviations' such as predilection for crime/theft, homosexuality, prostitution or drug/alcohol addiction and insanity, and has found some of its most refined forms in the developments of phrenology in the nineteenth century (Kemp and Wallace, 2000). To think of another example, in extreme Nazi or other racist ideologies non-conformity to the imposed body standard in terms of gender, ethnicity, class and so on has been seen as the source of perceived intellectual and moral inferiority of entire groups, communities and societies (Urla and Terry, 1995: 5). This concept of deviance can be related to Goffman's notion of *stigma*, that is 'an undesired differentness from what we had anticipated' (Goffman, 1997 [1963]: 74).

The fear of the *deviant* body implies and, in fact, can only be made meaningful in relation to the *ideal*, *desirable* and *normal* body. Of course, the ideal/idealised image of the body is not given, same and unchanging for all people, and at all times. Just as individuals' identities, self-perceptions, other-representations, and so on, are flexible, changeable and multiplex, so are the representations of the 'ideal' body. However, I suggest that at any given time in a specific community (be it a social, gender, professional, or any other group), there are certain well-recognised and accepted principles on which the idea of an ideal body is based. The discursive and/or visual representations of such ideal bodies are constituted by and constitutive of the power relations operating within the community.

The preoccupation with the *ideal vs. deviant* bodies has further links with power. Douglas (1996) argues that because the body can be used as a symbol of any bounded system, such as society, negotiating the margins of bodily acceptability can be indicative of negotiating the margins of society, and the shifting of these margins may have consequences for the centres of power. This can explain our fear of, and at the same time fascination with, 'freaks', 'monsters', 'cyborgs', 'aliens', and so on (Eubanks, 1996). Yet, our fascination with monsters *et al.* has also a more personal dimension. Shildrick (2002) argues that 'monsters', that is the excluded bodies that fail to conform to any corporeal norm, may sometimes turn up in our own self-perceptions. Instead of remaining at the outer regions of our embodied selves, they may at times reflect aspects of our own subjectivities, creating uncertainties and anxieties of our self-perception and self-identification (see also Stafford, 1991).

The aim of this chapter is, then, to analyse the *Naked* interviews to identify the areas invoked by the interviewees, in which they see their bodies conforming to or deviating from the perceived, if elusive, 'norm'. My focus here is on two specific categories in terms of which the interviewees invoke the ideal body image in relation to self: *age* and *gender/sexuality*. Because of space limitations, I do not discuss here other areas that provide other frames for discussing the body in *Naked*, for example *health and illness, ethnicity,* the body as a source of *physical and material capital, self-presentation, Significant Other's body, parenthood, freedom, death and dying.* Certainly, all these areas overlap to a great extent and I will touch upon many of them in the discussion below, but the two chosen for discussion here appear to be the dominant ones in the programme.

Age

By far the most frequent aspect of self-identity and self-reference invoked in the discourses of the body in *Naked* is the category of age: growing up, maturing and ageing. As has been mentioned before, the four parts of *Naked* take their titles from and focus on age-related issues. It is not hard to notice that the accepted age-related norm here is being in one's prime, whereas, other things being equal, puberty, middle-age and old age are anxiety-provoking or downright undesirable. The first part, titled 'Eighteen 'till I Die', deals with 'middle age'.

The opening off-camera interview suggests that, especially with regard to the category 'middle age', chronological age loses importance in projecting a self-identity, while contextual age, based on how one's body *feels* or *looks* can be a more readily accepted or preferred indicator of one's *age*:

Extract 8.1 [1]
M: I see myself sort of maturing (.) gracefully towards middle age (.) I'm (breathes) uh forty-two is (2.0) age is difficult it's very subjective I mean when I was sixteen (breathes) I probably thought forty-two was ancient whereas now I still feel as Bryan Adams would say you know eighteen till I die

Featherstone and Hepworth (1991) argue that the social and lifestyle developments of the last few decades have led to the radical changes in perceptions and organisation of individuals' (especially middle-class) lifecourses, such as relative blurring of boundaries between life stages and movement toward a uni-age style ('children are becoming more adult-like and adults more childlike' [Featherstone and Hepworth, 1991: 372]). These authors further suggest that the gradual decline of the significance of age-grading seems to be responsible for the growing resistance to the notion of 'middle-age', the term 'mid-life' being preferred in its place and stretching from anywhere in the mid-thirties to the early sixties or even beyond that chronological age.

M in Extract 8.1 identifies his chronological age ('forty-two'), but does not consider himself to be 'middle-aged', only 'maturing (.) gracefully toward middle age', the implication being that he is *young*. M is here picking his words from the available cultural scripts on ageing, which circulate in various domains, for example over 50s dating ads (Coupland, 2000) where 'maturing' is a common euphemism for 'ageing'. He *feels* youthful, and he invokes youthfulness by a reference to a pop idol: admittedly an ageing pop idol, but for many fans of 40 and over, a number of 50+/60+ pop stars such as Tina Turner, Mick Jagger, David Bowie, and so on, remain 'young for their age' and as such desirable points of reference in their own (fans') age self-identification.

However, even more importantly, it should be noted that in Extract 8.1, which opens the first programme and thus the entire series, the discussion of 'age' replaces the discussion of the 'body'. The latter is not mentioned explicitly, which indicates to what extent talk about age-related processes has become synonymous with discussing one's body.

In the next extract, the speaker does not explicitly claim the status of a young person for herself. She identifies her age at 'seventy', but she voices a sentiment, not unlike the one raised in Extract 8.1, that there is a frequent conflict between one's self-perception as young and advanced chronological age:

Extract 8.2 [4]

F: the whole process (.) I think is awful (laughs) (.) and the sad thing about being old is (.) you might feel twenty one (.) laughing joking (.) but I realise (.) no (.) I'm seventy years of age

F starts by complaining about the process of ageing, which she thinks 'is awful'. But whereas the listener may then expect a series of painful self-disclosures about poor health, loneliness, dependency, and so on, which are frequently associated with old age (Coupland *et al.*, 1991), the speaker laughs briefly, which prefaces a rather atypical account of what it is to be in old age, the incompatibility of chronological age with biological age: 'you might feel twenty-one laughing joking but I realise no I'm seventy years of age'. F creates a subversive image of an old person in relation to the dominant stereotype: instead of feeling poorly and being miserable, she positions herself as if she was young 'laughing joking'. Here, as in Extract 8.1, chronological age is invoked as an objective characteristic, but is subverted by a claim to the membership of the 'uni-age' group. Interestingly, extreme youth (eighteen to early twenties) is construed in the above two extracts (and indeed by other interviewees) as the archetype for that group. This, then, may be seen as the emerging 'norm' for the interviewees' self-perceptions, whereas advancing chronological age is inevitably associated with deviation from this norm.

Consistent with Featherstone and Hepworth's (1991) observations, most fears and anxieties voiced in *Naked* have to do with the loss of control over one's body, loss of motor and physiological flexibility, physical fitness and interpersonal skills owing to the malfunctioning body (including loss of appeal, desirability, or appreciation by others), and, ultimately, with death and dying. All of these themes are more or less explicitly present in the following extract(s) from an extended interview with a 'middle-aged' couple in the first episode of *Naked*:

Extract 8.3a [1]

M: I've got a vivid memory of um outside of the house I was (.) coming down off the roof and I went on to the the wall round the side of the house there (.) which is only five foot six in old money I suppose you know a meter and a half something like that (.) and I leapt off now I'd been up and down there quite a lot while we were renovating the property (.) and I hadn't been on that wall for a while and I leapt off and I hit the ground (F: laughs) and (.) it was just like somebody had whacked me on the bottom of my feet with a hammer there was just no bounce in the legs and it was one day it came as a hell of a shock you know and I just went whack oh no my knees didn't give [F: mhm:] you know everything had sort of stopped moving

Extract 8.3b [1]

M: nobody tells you about these things when you're young you know I was about five foot nine and a half when I was at my peak and I'm down to what not five foot nine now if you shrink if you're the same weight you look thicker because of course you're compressing (.) and that's why you tend to have this sort of middle age look about you (.) one of those unfair things again

Extract 8.3c [1]

M: there are other problems with (.) with ageing which are not obvious and one of those is that (.) you no longer become somebody which would turn somebody else's head as you walk down the street you still feel you're young you see so your eyes are looking out at a young person (.) all the young people go past and all they see is some old person waddling up the road (.) I suppose late thirties was the first time I noticed that sort of thing happen to me and it it's strange it's almost like being totally invisible except that they don't walk into you

Extract 8.3d [1]

Q: do you think you look the age that you are?

F: no: I don't think so I don't think that I look fifty ha ha I wasn't gonna say that but I don't think [M laughs] I do (clears her throat) I don't think I look <u>that</u> old (laughs) most people when they meet me don't think I am but then again you know face lift and stuff like that I'm I'm bound not to and uh

Q: what have you both had done tell me

F: well I've had face-lift upper and lower eyes I've ha:d um upper lip augmentation full face laser: (.) I've had what else have I had done I've had an uplift an:d (softly) liposuction (.) (softly) on my tummy (.) (normal volume) quite a lot really (.) bit bionic (laughs)

M: =is a bit yeah

Q: no wonder you look younger than you are

F: that's right cheat (.) why not? [to M] go ahead what have you had done?

M: I've had my nails done

F: (laughs) no tell the truth

M: I've had a face lift (.) and my lower eyes and my nose

Throughout the above four extracts, M and F identify a number of 'problems' their and other people's bodies inevitably experience while entering middle-age: absence of physical fitness (Extract 8.3a), changed body shape (Extract 8.3b), lack of attractiveness (Extract 8.3c). All these issues are presented as if they were the result of unexpected, sudden, shocking, strange and unfair loss, failure or departure from a comfortable and desirable state of being 'young'.

Extract 8.3d offers a brief insight into how F and M deal with the identified problems of their (middle-)ageing bodies. Prompted by the interviewer's question 'do you think you look the age that you are?', F engages in the discussion of how she and her partner resist the effects of ageing. A typical strategy is the concealment of chronological age. In providing her answer to Q, F reveals her chronological age: 'I don't think that I look fifty ha ha I wasn't gonna say that but I don't think [M laughs] I do (clears her throat) I don't think I look <u>that</u> old'. In providing this answer, F indicates that revealing one's chronological age is a cultural taboo; however, without doing so, she would not have been able to make her point of *not* looking her age convincingly. What we have here then is an admission of deviance (being 50 years old), in order to assure normalcy (not looking that old).

F's self-proclaimed not looking '<u>that</u> old' is further identified as inevitable because of her deliberate efforts to look 'young': 'face lift and stuff like that'. In fact, we get a fairly detailed account of F's (and M's) plastic surgery procedures (see Extract 8.3d). Additionally, the programme viewers can see numerous shots of F and M exercising extensively (which is probably what F refers to as 'stuff like that' in 'face lift and stuff like that').

Thus, a combination of keeping one's body in shape, plastic surgery, concealment of one's chronological age, and so on, are all voiced here as legitimate means of subverting old age and its effects on one's body. The exchange between Q and F: 'no wonder you look younger than you are / that's right cheat (.) why not', is indicative of F's discursive resource, which seems to have filtered to private discourses of the body from commercial/advertising discourses, in which using certain creams, for example, brings the promise of 'stopping the ageing process'. In such advertisements and in F's discourse, looking young is equated with being young (see Coupland and Hepworth, this volume).

By far the most frequent association of chronological ageing in *Naked* is with overall physical/aesthetic deterioration. As in the next extract, for example, time becomes identified as the sole factor and the identifying feature responsible for the body becoming what it ought not to be:

Extract 8.4 [1]

F: if I'm in the bath and I'm looking at my body I really don't like it (.) to be perfectly honest (.) it's almost like it was when I was going through puberty and I think menopause and puberty are very similar (1.0) when when you're in puberty you suddenly get (.) these bumps and (.) curves and (.) you don't quite know how to handle them and it's the same with ageing (1.0) you suddenly see yourself in the bath and the once perfect little bust that you had and the nipples just stoop

up on end and now they kind of fall a little down and (.)
instead of standing upright they kind of spread

In Extract 8.4, time is slotted into three compartments: 'puberty';
'menopause'; and the sexually attractive time in-between of 'the once
perfect little bust that you had and the nipples just stoop up on end'.
Interestingly, puberty and menopause appear to invoke similar references of F's dislike for her body and the declaration of not knowing
how to 'handle' it (on discourses of the menopause, see Coupland and
Williams, 2002; see also discussion of Extract 8.16 below). As is clear
from Extract 8.4, a crucial factor in accepting one's body (and self) is
related to the feeling of sexual attractiveness (see also Extracts 8.3a, 8.9
and next Section).

Likewise, the speaker in Extract 8.5 defines being in one's prime as
the time between puberty and old age (possibly menopause?):

Extract 8.5 [2]

F: I suppose you are in the prime of your life aren't you when (.)
      you when you're about twenty because you've gone past that
      adolescent puppy-fat stage and you're not quite the wrinkled
      (.) old geezer stage so you look like you're gonna look for the
      rest of your life but just without those wrinkles and the the
      (breathes) cellulite and nasty things like that

F in Extract 8.5 defines being 'in the prime of your life' as a well-
established period of one's life-cycle contrasted with two others: first,
'that adolescent puppy-fat stage', and second, 'the wrinkled (.) old
geezer stage'. In these cases, the inadequacy of the body is invoked as
an undesirable sign of immaturity (puppy-fat) and ageing (wrinkles,
cellulite), respectively. Not unlike F in Extract 8.4, the speaker here discusses her body as somewhat deviant or problematic before and after
reaching one's/her *prime*. In other words, the body grows out of its
adolescent inadequacies and then slips into those of the middle and
old age.

It is interesting to note that the 'mature' look of being in one's
prime is also treated in Extract 8.5 as some kind of *definitive* look of a
person: 'you look like you're gonna look for the rest of your life'. This
suggests reaching the self-perception of a well-formed, well-defined,
embodied self that will remain recognisable till the end of one's life
but inevitably will be damaged by the attributes of old age 'wrinkles
and the the (breathes) cellulite and nasty things like that'. Reaching

perfection brings with itself the promise of degeneration and decline; the norm defines the deviation, and vice versa.

Both Extracts 8.4 and 8.5 suggest, then, that an ideal body is not something one is born with. Unlike most manufactured goods, which are perfect only when they are (*brand*) new (or 'as new'), the body grows out of an imperfection into an *ideal*, and then starts sliding into another imperfection. The first part of this trajectory has been enshrined in Western literary tradition in the story of the ugly duckling (see also Extract 8.9).

In the Introduction, I suggested that some 'lay' discourses of the body may be informed by 'expert' ones. The next extract offers an overt exemplification of this influence. Note how in contrast to the previous extracts, in which bodies were positioned as part of the speakers' subjectivities, this example objectifies the body:

Extract 8.6 [1]

F: I had it explained to me by a physiotherapist that as you get older and you lose muscle tone in your diaphragm muscles your internal organs all do tend to move downwards a bit so it pushes your stomach out so that it looks bigger

This speaker's opinion appears to be informed by scientific/medical discourse ('I had it explained to me by a physiotherapist'), which seems to legitimise the changes of her body's size and shape: losing muscle, sagging and getting bigger. As we watch F's naked torso from the side, she speaks of her body as if giving an account of it to someone else: 'you lose muscle tone in your diaphragm muscles', 'your internal organs', 'your stomach'. The inevitability of such changes are not commented on negatively as in the previous two extracts, although it is clear that the speaker's (or anyone else's) body shape 'as you get older' needs an explanation or rationalisation in order not to be perceived as deviant.

Some interviewees equate the inevitability of the loss of a normative body with age but do not necessarily express any overt negativity or need to justify this process. As the speaker in the next extract states, the past is different from the present, and in terms of his body change, it has simply become 'fat':

Extract 8.7 [1]

M: I had six muscles three here and three there [point to his stomach] and they were all separated one here I can still feel a little bit and another one there and another one there in the shape of pyramid (.) and it looked exactly like a body builder but nothing else you know and now you know it is too fat you know I can feel you know they say if you pinch that [pinches the skin on his stomach] and if it goes more than a half an inch that means you're really fat I I am more than two inches I must be really fat yeah

Being 'fat' here is spoken about in a very matter-of-fact way. The speaker refers to lay discourses of assessing fatness by pinching the skin on one's stomach, and reports on having exceeded the fat threshold by about 'two inches'. There is only an implicit reference to the negative image of a fat body, and the speaker invokes it by contrasting being 'too fat' *now* with the shape of his body in the past: 'I had six muscles three here and three there ... in the shape of pyramid (.) and it looked exactly like a body builder'.

As has been suggested above, the inevitability of body change is also expected and accepted at a relatively young age – adolescence, which is seen as a passing stage, and passing on to something better (one's prime):

Extract 8.8 [3]
Two young teenage females.
F1:   if you think about it (.) you imagine all these little things running around your body making (.) like chiseling away or
F2:   yeah pressing buttons ((unclear))=
F1:   =to make things grow=
F2:   =skin making spots
F1:   yeah and you know it's like a bit freaky sometimes because um (.) you imagine these things making all these things happen and you like you just want to (.) exterminate them (.) go stop it and=
F1:   umm
F2:   =cause all of a sudden you start springing out here and spring out there and there and there and there's and it's like (.) these little (.) hormone bacteria things are running around your body trying to make it all happen

Extract 8.8 makes it clear that adolescence is treated as a time that is uncomfortable ('freaky'), if necessary and transient. Both speakers seem to dissociate themselves from their bodies, or more specifically, from the processes which their bodies are undergoing, which are attributed to various external agents inside their bodies: 'little things running round your body', 'these things', 'hormone bacteria things'. The adolescent body is further represented here as if it was invaded by all these external agents and 'chiseling away', 'pressing buttons', 'making all these things happen', 'running around your body trying to make it all happen'. There is a clear analogy here between the way the adolescent body is discussed and the reification of disease, which 'many people conceive of germs and of malevolent entities residing in the body' (Gwyn, 2002: 32–3). And just as F1 in Extract 8.8 talks about her desire to 'exterminate' 'these things', cleaning the body of unwanted, alien influences is how treatment of illness is often conceptualised. Gwyn states:

> Expulsion of germs from the urinary tract and from the bowels is considered by Helman (1978) in his study of folk beliefs in a London suburb. He treats expulsion as one of three ways to deal with the invasive *it* in its guise as a 'Germ', the other two being starvation (as in the folk saying 'feed a cold, starve a fever') and killing the germ *in situ*, by means of antibiotics.
>
> (Gwyn, 2002: 21)

As the passing time is concerned, then, there is a degree of fatalism present in most interviewees' discussions of their bodies, especially when some aspect of bodily deviance is mentioned. For a smaller number of interviewees, however, getting the 'perfect' body, or defending the body from the negative effects of ageing, is an active project in which little is left to chance so that the body can conform to the person's positive auto-stereotype. Such is the case of a 'man in his prime', interviewed in segment 2 of *Naked*. M is a professional entertainer in his late twenties/early thirties:

Extract 8.9 [2]

M: I was definitely not (.) born with this body I have worked really really hard I was really really skinny for a long long time (.) too long just like just you know and I could never pull a girl (.) just could not get a girl no chance (.) cause I was just this tall (.) puny geezer d'you know what I mean I was like fifteen or something and just couldn't get girls don't know maybe I was just a ugly duckling (laughs) (.) and maybe grew up to a swan

Here, the speaker in his 'prime' contrasts two periods of his life: his adolescence and the present, and two corresponding body images: the inadequate 'really skinny' body when he was 15 years old, and the fully acceptable, muscular body of today. The two body images are not contrasted simply in terms of what M looked like in the past and now, but predominantly in terms of what he (his body) was/is capable of doing. The adolescent 'skinny' body was not only disproportionate: 'too long', 'tall (.) puny geezer', 'ugly duckling', but its owner was sexually unappealing and unable to attract the attention of females: 'I could never pull a girl (.) just could not get a girl no chance'. It is implied that the 'swan'-like, fit body that M proudly displays in front of the camera is capable of attracting numerous sexual partners.

There is another reason why maintaining M's body in perfect order is important to him. A little later in the interview he describes in some detail how he uses his body to make a living:

Extract 8.10 [2]
M: if I was to stop training (.) where would my wages come from (.) body painting modelling stripping all's all revolves around body body body (.) my body is definitely my money

Thus, it is not only that M needs his body to remain attractive to secure his access to sexual partners. He needs to carry on 'training' to maintain it in good shape for economic gain. In fact, M describes the commodification of his body as quite successful:

Extract 8.11 [2]
M: I left school when I was sixteen (.) um didn't have a brilliant education at all and when I look back on how I started to use my body to make a living (1.0) I've got two houses and a BMW and money in the bank and nobody's given me anything two houses and a BMW and money in the bank isn't bad (.) you know

But even though M appears to be self-satisfied with what his body is like now compared to what it was like in his adolescence (Extract 8.9), and how it earns him a comfortable living (Extracts 8.10 and 8.11), he is far from seeing his body as *perfect*.

Extract 8.12 [2]
Q: do you think that your body is the best it could ever be?

M: no (1.0) no no no I need to lose about another 5 or 6 pounds
     I'd say maybe (laughs) and then maybe I'll be happy with it or
     but then am I ever going to be happy with it
Q: where are you going to lose 5 or 6 pounds from?
M: I can lose it I can lose it there's a bit there's a few bits you
     just don't know where it is (1.0) (laughing) don't be dirty
     (laughs)

The 'need' to lose weight on the part of M, who is otherwise
expressly satisfied with his body image (see Extract 8.9), may be an
unreasonable proposition even for him (note the frequent laughter
with which he talks about this in Extract 8.12). But this may also be
an expression of a widespread fear of humans to lose (or never be
able to attain) a perfect body they crave, or to ward off the
inevitable: deterioration of one's body, death and decay, for as long
as possible.

So far, I have examined several extracts from *Naked*, in which the
interviewees expressed various beliefs and attitudes towards their
bodies in relation to ageing. The dominant three themes to have
emerged so far are as follows:

1.   A person's life-cycle is marked by self-conceptualisations of one's
     body as inadequate or deviant during one's adolescence and in
     later stages of life described as middle-age, old-age, menopause,
     which contrasts with the acceptable/ideal body image in one's
     'prime'. While in his/her prime, the body is a 'true' representation
     of self; life-span can be seen as a person's working towards achiev-
     ing the acceptable/true body image, battling to maintain it, and
     eventually losing it to old age.
2.   The body can be transformed from the state of deviance to nor-
     malcy either through 'work' or as part of natural development
     through the working of time. The latter perception works also in
     the other direction, from normalcy to deviance, namely after one's
     prime, the body takes its course towards deterioration. More work
     and effort (for example investing in plastic surgery, physical exer-
     cise) may be used to adhere to the norm of an ideal body for
     longer.
3.   An ideal or acceptable body is a prerequisite to acquiring and sus-
     taining a healthy sex life.

This last point is the focus of the next section.

Gender and sexuality

As evolutionary scientists have argued for a long time, the main reason for our existence is reproduction. Regardless of whether this view is true or not, it is a truism to observe that sexual activities, leading to reproduction or not, are highly prized and associated with rewards and gratification. (I disregard such pathological manifestations of sexual activity as rape and paedophilia.) It is not surprising, then, to find in the data numerous references orienting interviewees' bodies to sex. In fact, sex is a salient feature of talk in all four episodes of *Naked*, which cut across all age-groups, starting in the youngest age-group represented in the programme – adolescents:

Extract 8.13 [3]
Two teenage boys.
M2: right (.) cause um we don't we boys don't wear make up right um (.) most boys don't wear make up
M1: (laughs)
M2: .hhh it's like there's not really things much things we can work with apart from our hair (.) you know and um (.) our hygiene and stuff (.) so we have to try and (.) maintain the best (.) thing possible (.) cause at this age it's mostly about girls I think like attracting girls (.) at this age
M2: yeah
M1: cause like your hormones are raging and everything
Q: how old are you
M1: fourteen
.
.
.
M1: everyday is a shower man (.) it's like
M2: yeah
M1: I have to have deodorant as well
M2: yeah deodorant that's a (exhales) major
M1: I hate b o
M2: and (.) chewing gum sometimes yeah=
M1: I hate bad breath
M2: =when you're going (.) away you going to need something because (.) all through the day (.) you not ne-necessarily going to be able to wash your brush your teeth twice a day so (.) if what do you call it (.) in the middle of the day you just take a chewing gum (.) chew it just helps to to just keep my breath fresh

M1: yeah

.

.

M1: the thing I like best about my appearance are my physical side (.) .hhh you know (.) muscles (.) my face (0.5) penis (.) um

M2: (laughing)

M1: (.) yeah=

Q: =why is penis important

M1: just the size of it cause

M2: hhh. too right

M1: if a girl finds out that you've got some little small sized penis like that size there

M2: yeah that's true cause you never hear a girl saying (.) oh I want a man with a small penis

M1: yeah you never [hear] it

M2: [you never] hear it man

M1: they want (.) full size

.

.

M1: I'd love to [have big] muscles

M2: [uh yeah]

M1: but I don't really have it (.) but I've started doing a little bit of weight training and so I should begin to put on some more weight soon so

M2: I can see my pack starting to develop a bit

M1: yeah yeah me too yeah

M2: and it's like (.) the older I feel I want to put on a bit of weight and then pump out a bit=

M1: yeah

M2: =but it's easier said but you know I feel that's what I want to do so that's what I am going to do

Q: why why do you want them to be bigger

M2: cause I like a more (.) broad bull look it's like=

M1: =yeah yeah when the girls look at you they look at your muscles=

[

M2:   yeah yeah it's true it's true

M1: =the whole how you carry your self =

M2: =it's true=

M1:   =and if you've got bigger muscles the easier the the chance
      that she's going that you can defend her in in difficulty or
      something like that

This extended extract is a vivid example of one of many direct formulations of the sexualised body in the programme. The two fourteen-
year-old boys discuss sex in great detail as the main reason for looking
after their bodies, 'cause at this age it's mostly about girls I think like
attracting girls (.) at this age', their grooming practices: taking a shower
every day, using deodorant, maintaining fresh breath (chewing gum),
and being expressly proud of certain physical characteristics: 'the thing
I like best about my appearance are my physical side (.) .hhh you know
(.) muscles (.) my face (0.5) penis (.) um'. Clearly, the three aspects of
the body mentioned by M1 here are highly gendered: 'muscles' have
clear associations with masculinity, 'face' is the prime part of the body,
which we use for person recognition, as well age and sex identification
(Bruce and Young, 1998), and, of course, the penis is the ultimate
symbol of masculinity. Thus, by striving to make their bodies fit into
the expected norm of attractiveness and conforming to the stereotyped
gender expectations, 'cause you never hear a girl saying (.) oh I want a
man with a small penis', 'if you've got bigger muscles the easier the the
chance that she's going that you can defend her in in difficulty or
something like that', M1 and M2 construe their bodies as primarily
sexual entities and/or with reference to stereotypically heterosexual
masculine characteristics (for example defenders of women).

Extract 8.13 has a number of similarities with Extract 8.8, in which
the two teenage girls engage in the exchange of cultural scripts about
ageing. Compare the following: 'these little (.) hormone bacteria things
are running around your body trying to make it all happen' (Extract
8.8); 'cause like your hormones are raging and everything' (Extract
8.13). In each of these two extracts, the speakers refer to biologically
driven bodily processes, although in Extract 8.13, the teenage boys link
them explicitly to their future, planned sexual activity.

The notion of the norm underlying the boys' body projects is manifested in their discussion of the positives in how their bodies are
shaped (see above) as well as what they find in need of improvement
and how they are going to achieve them: 'I'd love to [have big] muscles
... but I don't really have it (.) but I've started doing a little bit of
weight training and so I should begin to put on some more weight
soon so', 'I can see my pack starting to develop a bit ... and it's like (.)
the older I feel I want to put on a bit of weight and then pump out a

bit'. These boys, then, orient to a specific image of an ideal body (note the amount of agreement in their descriptions of its salient features), and express a determination in carrying out their body projects: 'but it's easier said but you know I feel that's what I want to do so that's what I am going to do'.

The *Naked* interviewees discuss sex with reference to a wide range of issues. Not surprisingly, the ability of one's body to engage in sex, or making an impression of sexual attractiveness, is a major theme. Maintaining sexual activity can be the source of concern, pride, anxiety and even a sufficient reason to undergo a painful operation: 'face lift and stuff like that'. Moreover, the spoken and visual discourse in the programme seems to focus on the differences rather than the similarities between the bodies of both sexes. Visually, the programme is replete with close-ups of female breasts, hips and buttocks, and male genitals and hairy chests.

A sense of sexual attractiveness resulting from the approbation of one's body image is the theme of the next extract, in which an ideal body is modelled after a recognisable pop icon's image:

Extract 8.14 [1]

F: I had uh breast enlargement about three years ago the incisions were made just under here it's a very painful operation but I consider it to be worth it I went in with a picture of Madonna and asked the surgeon for her boobs and now I have them and I'm delighted with them

As far as F in Extract 8.14 claims self-confidence related to an improved body image, M in Extract 8.15 voices concern that he (and most other men) cannot appear sexually attractive to women:

Extract 8.15 [1]

M: there is a size of penis which for most women ah will give them <u>maximum</u> satisfaction the impression I'm under is that that size amounts to about seven to eight inches which leaves the average male completely up the swanny without a paddle

Thus, the body in *Naked* is set against a specific *gendered* norm. Breast size and shape (Extract 8.14) and penis size (Extract 8.15) can be seen as typical, gender-specific concerns of women and men, respectively (or vice versa!), and the last two extracts are quite representative of many interviewees in *Naked* referring to their bodies by focusing on the most frequently gendered body parts. In doing so, they tend to invoke the idea of fitting (or not) to a clearly defined norm: 'I went in with a picture of Madonna and asked the surgeon for her boobs'. Furthermore, Extract 8.15, as well as Extract 8.16 below, can be viewed as pathologising the body with very tangible consequences for the self-perception and well-being of the interviewee. F in Extract 8.16 is the same person as F in Extract 8.4 talking about her 'lost' perfect body owing to menopause. In another part of the interview, her chronological age is identified as 54.

Extract 8.16 [1]

F: now I don't feel physical any more because (.) the thought of perhaps disappointing someone [Q: hmm] when you say take your clothes off [Q: hmm] and and you don't look the way you used to and I suppose I'm just (.) thinking that someone would be disappointed but they wouldn't want to tell me

In the above extract, F confesses complete celibacy as a result of her negative auto-stereotype. Here, the ageing body is not contrasted with some kind of generic body ideal, or that of a pop icon, but with the way F used to look in the past, and with the implication of her past active sex life. In this sense, this extract is reminiscent of Extract 8.5, in which the interviewee prepares herself and others for her altered body image to be destroyed by wrinkles, cellulite and other 'nasty things like that'. In relation to this and other extracts from this interview, it is useful to quote Lupton's (1996) observation:

> The meaning around the ageing feminine body in both popular and medical discourses centres around the loss of attractiveness, fertility and function. Physical appearance is integral to feminine subjectivity in Western societies. The middle-aged and older woman's body is typically portrayed as asexual and undesirable, and the less of youth and sexual attractiveness is experienced as a major source of alienation and anxiety for many women, particularly those who have derived a sense of power and satisfaction from their sexual attractiveness.
>
> (Lupton, 1996: 92)

In the fourth segment of *Naked*, which deals with the body in later life, the mention of sex/sexuality and age may have the most painful recollections for the interviewees, especially when one has to admit that his or her sex life is confined to the past, which is usually (for males) a euphemism for disclosing one's impotence. This is when the bodily experience of old age comes to the fore, and the definitive cessation of sexual activity appears to be inevitable. This point is made explicitly in the following extract:

Extract 8.17 [4]

M:　I still need sex (.) but unfortunately it <u>has</u> gone (.) not like (0.5) little bit (.) it (.) disappeared (.) well the thoughts there (.) it's there all the time (laughs) but it don't w- you know it uh doesn't happen (.) you know (.) it's like saying well I want to go out in a car but (.) I ain't got a car

Here M expresses a longing for sex in the same way other people may express a longing for their good looks from their youth. M implies quite vividly the state of his impotence, which makes sex a thing of the past for him and totally unattainable. But not all 'old' people find sex to be unavailable because of impotence. In the next extract, M, who identifies himself in the interview as being 'almost' 85, challenges the view of an 'old' body as asexual.

Extract 8.18 [4]

M:　obviously at my age I could not expect to (.) attract people as I might have been able to (.) when I was very much younger (.) I'm not impotent but uh obviously it's harder (0.5) and my sexual urges are still quite strong (0.5) and if (.) I didn't have (.) this very absorbing activity with my mind I love writing my book uh then I might be uh quite unhappy (2.0) in other respects (.) I can (.) I <u>walk</u> more now than I used to when I was (.) much younger (.) I don't fee:l uh winding down

M in Extract 8.18 is more like F in Extract 8.16 rather than M in Extract 8.17. He talks here of his body posing a problem in attracting sexual partners rather than his inability to engage in sex. Yet, another older person (of undisclosed age) claims not to miss sex at all and prefers other physical pleasures:

Extract 8.19 [4]

F:　sex to me is ((unclear)) (.) I don't bother with it (.) waste of time (.) I'd sooner have a-a nice cup of tea (.) a nice cheese sandwich and a pickled onion

The last three quotes cited above (Extract 8.17–19) attest to the common stereotype that old people do not engage in sex because they can't, don't want to, or because their potential partners would not find them attractive enough to do so. This is probably a false stereotype and there are older people appearing in the programme who at least imply that they engage in sex. But the fear of old age and the associated changes in one's body – wrinkling, sagging, thinning hair, and so on – is quite tangible in interviewees of almost all ages. And it is not simply the fear of 'looking old' but the fear of not looking attractive, and hence, losing access to sex.

Although several interviewees in *Naked* raise their anxieties about losing their sexual attractiveness or desire for sex, various others appear to define their bodies positively with reference to their active sexual lifestyles. Apparently, sexual fulfilment can override individuals' concerns with the ageing process and body shape. Thus, to a great extent, *Naked* is a celebration of sex and the sexualised body.

Extract 8.20 [1]

M: it's difficult to: um (.) to put into words what it feels to be middle age I think I'm in a reasonably good nick for a forty year old as far as most gay men are concerned you're probably over the hill but I don't think I am over the hill not by any stretch of imagination

Extract 8.21 [1]

F: going into the porn industry I've learnt a lot about myself my sexuality to be so in touch with your body and and find out the amount of power that you have within I guess you could say I'm having my wonder years in my forties

As the above two extracts suggest, being sexually active and free to explore one's sexuality is a source of reassurance, self-confidence and self-satisfaction. Although obviously positive self-image may depend on several different factors (for example relative wealth, intellectual achievement, and so on), the acceptance of one's body image by self, one's partner and others, is an important aspect of developing self-respect and self-confidence. By linking self-confidence to sexual activity, and the latter to the notion of 'young age', we can find reinforcement for the observations that ceasing to maintain sexual attractiveness is equated with laziness, low self-esteem and even low moral ground (Featherstone, 1991). The interviewees in *Naked* seem to reinforce such views, probably taking their cue from contemporary mass media's obsession with the cult of young age and sex.

Just as an individual's body image may affect his/her relationships with others, the opposite is also true. In the following extract, a couple after thirteen years of marriage discuss their relationship in relation to the fluctuating body weight and image of F:

Extract 8.22 [2]

F: I was so enamoured with having a a new born baby anyway that my body really took second place I became (.) virtually asexual and that was a a real low point in my (.) relationship with Trevor I just put on a ton of weight and mainly to: avoid any kind of (.) sexual attention

I':ve spent many many years battling with this dichotomy of how do you be (.) a mother and a lover at the same time you've used the the sa- self same parts of your body to bring life into the world to feed it and nurture it how do you then claim it back in order to to become (.) a sexually active (.) <u>fulfilled</u> woman

M: Sarah's body (1.0) contains no mysteries (.) after thirteen years but (.) there are (.) so many fascinating places to go it's like (.) living in a big town as opposed to a small village (.) you know everywhere but you still want to go there

F: my husband Trevor has been the the m<u>ost</u> ardent fan of my body throughout the last thirteen years (.) it's very difficult to (.) uh retain low self esteem when you have someone telling you day in day out how wonderful you are (.) it's very difficult to uh like yourself and hate your body (.) I would say impossible

The aesthetics of F's (Sarah's) body fits the ideal of Rubens's women rather than that of contemporary fashion magazines. And although F's partner M (Trevor) is happy to follow Rubens's rather than David Bailey's taste in the portrayal of the female body, the path towards his partner's self-acceptance was long and fraught with difficulty. At present, F may still think of herself as 'fat', but she seems to have come to terms with her body image in part thanks to M's construal of her body as, paraphrasing, a fascinating place to go to over and over again.

Sarah appears to have completed her quest for the perfect body, that is she has accepted her own: 'it's very difficult to (.) uh retain low self esteem when you have someone telling you day in day out how wonderful you are', and this has had a positive effect on her self-perception overall: 'I started to like my self (.) a great deal more when I started coming to terms with the body that I have'. Sadly, many other interviewees in *Naked* may never finish their quest for the perfect body and a harmonious relationship between self and body.

In sum, as presented in *Naked*, the normative body is a sexually functioning one and the aestheticisation of the body is constructed primarily as a concern for interpersonal attractiveness and sexual gratification of self and/or (significant) other. Interestingly, the programme foregrounds the interviewees' concern with sex and old age much more than, for example, health. If mentioned at all, issues such as excercising and healthy diet are discussed more in terms of their merits for the aesthetics of one's body rather than one's physical well-being.

Conclusion

In *Naked*, talk of the ideal *vs.* deviant body is present or implied virtually throughout the entire programme in all interviews. The ideal body is referred to in terms of an unattainable or lost dream, a mythical quest, a realistic prospect, or, indeed, a desirable current state. Although, as mentioned in the Introduction, other themes were also discussed by the interviewees, the main ones are age, gender and sexuality. These were the concepts to which I have predominantly related the discussion of norm and deviance in the discursive self-presentations of the body.

A common denominator available for the above discussion can be found in Shilling's (1993) dualistic view of the body as a biological and social entity. The discourse emerging from *Naked* can be seen as performing a dual (though interlinked) role. First, it allows individuals to voice their experiences of the body in relation to their physicality, sensuality and fitness, and second, it allows them to produce socially desirable and competing versions of their bodies for self and other. Thus, discourse becomes a site of the interface between the biological and social forces that shape bodies, and it is also a site of ideological struggle between the projected body image clashing with the body of one's (or others') dominant perceptions and/or expectations.

In this vein, although most of the discourses in *Naked* seem to conform to the dominant ideologies of the body which conceptualise the normative body as 'young', 'attractive', 'sexualised', and so on, a number of participants in the programme appear to subvert and challenge these notions. The following two extracts are examples of such subversive work with regard to defying the effect of old age on one's body (23) and finding sexual fulfilment in a body that does not conform to the 'slim' ideal (24):

Extract 8.23 [4]

M: it's slowed down but it's still nice it's:: probably like driving a really fast car and then later on you get a little slow car and you start looking at the birds and the countryside and hedges and you think well I am not going as fast as I used to but the scenery is much better you know

Extract 8.24 [2]

F: I was surprised (.) when my figure was fuller at how erotic it felt how how nice it felt to be voluptuous (2) it was a shock actually because I always thought (.) I'd wanted to be slim and that this was sexy to be slim but there's something much more erotic about being bigger and voluptuous

Another man (in Programme 4) argues that old age is an 'achievement' and it brings 'respect'; he says: 'old age is a privilege in life'.

Whether by accepting or challenging the normative view of the body (*vs.* the pathologised/stigmatised view), all the interviewees seem to invoke the dichotomy of norm *vs.* deviation in talking about their bodies. The interviewees range between characterising their bodies as satisfactory enough to be the locus of their authentic selves, or adequate representations of their selves, and describing their bodies as inappropriate or fraudulent frames hiding their 'true' personas (see Jaworski in preparation for a more detailed discussion of these issues). Thus, it is hoped that this chapter manages to reinforce the major theme of this volume by arguing that the body and selfhood are intimately interrelated and largely mediated by spoken discourse.

Acknowledgements

I thank Justine Coupland for useful comments on earlier incarnations of this chapter. I am grateful to Susan Hogben for the transcripts and to the Cardiff Centre for Language and Communication for financial assistance in the preparation of this chapter.

Transcription Conventions

[1], [2], [3], [4] – numbers in square brackets in extract headings indicate which episode the extract is from.

[– overlapping speech

= – contiguous speech

: – lengthening

(.) – brief pause

(1.0) – pause of about 1 second

.hhh – audible in-breath

hhh. – audible out-breath

<u>maximum</u> – extra stress

sa- – incomplete word

(breathes) – other paralinguistic and non-verbal information

[hear] – unclear word, best guess

((unclear)) – unclear text

vertical stops – text missing

References

Beck, Ulrich (1992) *Risk Society: Towards a New Modernity*. London: Sage.

Beck, Ulrich (1994) 'The Reinvention of Politics: Towards a Theory of Reflexive Modernization'. In Ulrich Beck, Anthony Giddens and S. Lash (eds) *Reflexive Modernization: Politics, Tradition and Aesthetics in the Modern Social Order*. Cambridge: Polity Press, 1–55.

Bruce, Vicki and Young, Andy (1998) *In the Eye of the Beholder: The Science of Face Perception*. Oxford: Oxford University Press.

Coupland, Justine (2000) 'Past the "Perfect Kind of Age"? Styling Selves and Relationships in Over-50s Dating Advertisements'. *Journal of Communication* 50.

Coupland, Justine and Williams, Angie (2002) 'Conflicting Discourses, Shifting Ideologies: Pharmaceutical, "Alternative" and Emancipatory Texts on the Menopause'. *Discourse & Society* 13.

Coupland, Nikolas, Coupland, Justine and Giles, Howard (1991) *Language, Society and the Elderly*. Oxford: Blackwell.

Douglas, Mary (1966) *Purity and Danger*. Baltimore: Penguin.

Edwards, Mark (1998) 'I Just Can't Bare It'. *The Sunday Times*, Culture, 22 November: 29.

Eubanks, Virginia (1996) 'Zones of Dither: Writing the Postmodern Body'. *Body & Society* 2(3): 73–88.

Featherstone, Mike (1991) 'The Body in Consumer Culture'. In Mike Featherstone, Mike Hepworth and Bryan S. Turner (eds) (1991) *The Body: Social Processes and Cultural Theory*. London: Sage, 170–96.

Featherstone, Mike and Mike Hepworth (1991) 'The Mask of Ageing and the Postmodern Life Course'. In Mike Featherstone, Mike Hepworth and Bryan S. Turner (eds) (1991) *The Body: Social Processes and Cultural Theory*. London: Sage, 371–89.

Foucault, Michel (1977) *Discipline and Punish: The Birth of the Prison.* Transl. A.M. Sheridan Smith. New York: Vintage Books.

Foucault, Michel (1979) *The History of Sexuality: An Introduction.* Transl. Robert Huxley. London: Penguin.

Giddens, Anthony (1990) *The Consequences of Modernity.* Cambridge: Polity Press.

Giddens, Anthony (1991) *Modernity and Self-Identity: Self and Society in the Late Modern Age.* Cambridge: Polity Press.

Goffman, Erving (1997) 'The Stigmatized Self'. In Charles Lemert and Ann Branman (eds) *The Goffman Reader.* Oxford: Blackwell. 73–79. [Originally published as *Stigma: Notes on the Management of Spoiled Identity.* Boston: Simon & Schuster (1963)]

Gwyn, Richard (2002) *Communicating Health and Illness.* London: Sage Publications.

Helman, C. (1978) '"Feed a Cold, Starve a Fever" – Folk Models of Infection in an English Suburban Community, and their Relation to Medical Treatment'. *Culture, Medicine and Psychiatry* 2: 107–37.

Jaworski, Adam. in preparation. 'The discursive construction of the self *vs.* body dichotomy'.

Joseph, Joe (1998) 'Revealing Programme, but is It Too Much?' 26 November, *The Times,* Review: 55.

Kemp, Martin and Wallace, Marina (2000) *Spectacular Bodies: The Art and Science of the Human Body from Leonardo to Now.* London: Hayward Gallery Publications and Berkeley: University of California Press.

Lupton, Deborah (1996) 'Constructing the Menopausal Body: the Discourses on Hormone replacement therapy'. *Body & Society* 2(1): 91–7.

Lupton, Deborah (2000) 'The Social Construction of Medicine and the Body'. In Gary I. Albert, Ray Fitzpatrick and Susan C. Scrimshaw (eds) *Handbook of Social Studies in Health and Medicine.* London: Sage, 50–63.

Lupton, Deborah and Tulloch, John (1998) 'The Adolescent "Unfinished Body", Reflexivity and HIV/AIDS Risk'. *Discourse & Society* 4(2): 19–34.

Midgley, Carol (1998) 'Gloomy Bennett Lets TV Cast Light on his Darkness'. *The Times,* 27 August: 9.

Shildrick, Margrit (2002) *Embodying the Monster: Encounters with the Vulnerable Self.* London: Sage.

Shilling, Chris (1993) *The Body and Social Theory.* London: Sage.

Stafford, Barbara Maria (1991) *Body Criticism: Imaging the Unseen in Enlightenment Art and Medicine.* Cambridge, MA: MIT Press.

Urla, Jacqueline and Terry, Jennifer (1995) 'Introduction: Mapping Embodied Deviance'. In Jennifer Terry and Jacqueline Urla (eds) *Deviant Bodies: Critical Perspectives on Difference in Scenic and Popular Culture.* Bloomington: Indiana University Press: 1–18.

9
Bodies Exposed: A Cross-cultural Semiotic Comparison of the 'Saunaland' in Germany and Britain

Ulrike Hanna Meinhof

Introduction

Germany and England share traditions of 'being naked' in public in movements such as Naturism and Nudism. But there are surprising major differences in the way the general public in both countries (re)present their (un-)clothed bodies in everyday leisure situations.

In contemporary Germany the adherence to Nudism of a tiny minority (FKK = Freikörperkultur: literally 'free body culture') does not explain the much more widespread pursuit of forms of leisure where nakedness in public is entirely taken for granted. 'Stripping off' in Germany may simply be the preferred, potentially illegal yet irrepressible, behaviour of some groups or individuals amongst others who remain safely dressed, as is the case on many free access beaches on the Baltic and North Sea, on lakes and even public centre-of-town parks such as the English Garden in Munich. Or being naked can be the (institutionally) correct form of 'un'-dress as is the case in saunas, be they private or public. The difference from English social behaviour in both, spontaneous as well as the institutionalised forms of nakedness, is so distinct that German visitors to England and English visitors to Germany are faced with something approaching a culture-shock.

My interest, in this chapter, lies in the institutional semiotics and commercial discourses of saunas in both countries – from the architectural layout to the instructions to (and behaviour of some of) its users. I will argue that taken in conjunction these 'discourses' amount to implicit or explicit constructions of the body as healthy, leisurely, sexy or illicit. My analysis will be based on data from several typical saunas in both countries and some of the connected texts about nakedness. I will try to draw some preliminary and highly generalised connections between attitudes to and discourses about the naked body in the UK and Germany on the one hand, and secondly, what, for want of a better phrase, I will call the semiotics of the sauna in both countries. My analysis will thus highlight the ways in which peoples' acculturated use of the rules and norms within each country is reflected in and confirmed by the various signs and presentational aspects of the respective saunas in both cultures.

On being naked in public

Let me begin with two anecdotes, both from a part of Germany where metropolitan life meets and sometimes clashes with Catholic Bavarian tradition. The place is Munich, the time is 1984.

Anecdote Number 1 begins with a letter to the editor of the liberal daily national but Munich-based newspaper *Süddeutsche Zeitung* (SZ) by a Herr Lorenz. This letter was written in reaction to a most spectacular hailstorm on 12 July 1984, which had showered several suburbs of the city with icy pebbles the size of small apples, killing cats and other small animals, shattering windows and damaging roofs, and making parked cars look as if they had been attacked by gunfire. On the SZ letter page, Herr Lorenz points out that this hailstorm was fitting punishment for all those naked people who were displaying themselves in public in the main public park right in the centre of Munich, the 'Englische Garten'. Following this original letter, the SZ was inundated with further letters, six of which it subsequently printed in a selection (SZ, 2 August 1984, p. 14). All these letter-writers expressed their great amusement at the suggestion that God's wrath had thus descended upon the naked of Munich. Two letters in particular were dripping with sarcasm, accusing God of having badly missed his target. The first of these two letters pointed out that the English Garden was long void of people before the hailstorm struck and, furthermore, was situated in a part of Munich rather less afflicted by the hailstorm than other areas which were not known for their parks with naked bodies. The other letter reminded the readers that God was well known for punishing through lightning but did not do too well in hitting his target. He points out that when God's wrath was awakened by the appointment of the then Bishop of York, he had also sent a coup of lightning to the Cathedral, but had missed the Bishop. And, similarly, the Munich hailstorm did not manage to damage any of the naked people in the Englische Garten.

Anecdote Number 2 takes us to a small pebbled beach in central Munich on the bank of the fast-flowing River Isar, which can only be reached by a very steep descent on a long metal ladder. The beach is difficult to get to – the ladder stops anyone who is not agile enough or who is scared of heights – but is not secluded from view for people on the opposite side of the river. Usually people sunbathe and swim there in the nude, though technically – just like in the Englische Garten nearby – full nudity is not legal, and technically, people could be arrested for causing a public nuisance. One hot summer day an older lady of about 60 years of age who was sunbathing there was approached by a young woman of about 20 years, and asked the following: 'Sag mal, kannste mir vielleicht eine von deinen Zigaretten schenken' (Hey, could you perhaps let me have one of your cigarettes) whereupon the older lady said in a very sharp tone: 'Was bilden Sie sich ein. Das kommt überhaupt nicht in Frage' (How can you imagine such a thing. There's no question of that.) Having accidentally overheard this exchange I interpreted its – to me surprisingly hostile-tone as follows: being nude together on this beach clearly did not create a bonding with the younger woman for the older one, which would have made the request for sharing a private resource, the cigarette, acceptable. The cigarette was therefore refused, the young woman rebuffed – end of story. Except that this explanation was incomplete: a moment later a friend of the older woman climbed down the ladder and was immediately told the story together with an explanation of why the woman had refused the request for the cigarette. It was, she said, that she had felt insulted by being addressed in the informal 'Du' by such a young whippersnapper, rather than the more formal 'Sie'.

What is the point about these two stories in the context of this chapter? The first instance shows, in my opinion, that the idea of nakedness in public, however much against the law it may be, could not possibly be constructed as sinful by the majority of readers of the *Süddeutsche Zeitung*. To them such a thought was ludicrous and worthy of mockery, and a great deal of fun at the poor original writer's expense ensued. The second instance is even more interesting. Being naked together and in public, namely violating a legal code, is fine but such violation does not automatically provide a bonding or in-groupedness which allows the violation of the sociolinguistic code. From the perspective of the older woman but not from that of the younger one this code would have called for the reciprocal formal mode of address between strangers – a 'Sie' – especially where there is a distinct age-gap. The implicit offer of solidarity – a reciprocal informal 'Du' – offered by the young to the older as one naked woman to another was neither recognised nor accepted as such by the older, and instead was interpreted as an insulting lack of respect for her. (See the classical and often reprinted paper by Brown and Gilman, 1960/1972.)

I would like to suggest that the ways in which nakedness appears and is being viewed in the specific settings of my two anecdotes – a public park or a stretch of beach by a river in Munich – point to something rather interesting about attitudes to the naked body amongst many Germans, of which the following three strike me as particularly significant. The experience of being naked in public:

1. is not constructed as an experience of shared brotherhood and sisterhood based on ideological bonding. It thus does not, or does no longer, resemble the movements of Naturism in Germany of the 1920s and 1930s, and it certainly does not resemble the institutionalised forms of Naturism in the UK or its remnants in the German Freikörperkultur – the 'free body culture' – all of which are heavily ideologised, and based on strict rules and norms of behaviour for a dedicated and inclusivist in-crowd of followers;

2. is not constructed as separatist in any other form either. Unlike, for example, the ageing membership of the Naturist movement it is not normally age-determined. Nor is it divided by class, gender or sexual practices (e.g., gay *vs.* heterosexual), since people of all kinds and orientation mix freely in the two areas in Munich that gave rise to the two anecdotes above. Again this is different from some institutionalised forms of nakedness on the few, often strongly sexually constructed nudist beaches in the UK (i.e., male and gay, as on the once highly controversial creation of a nudist beach in Brighton, and the anxiety this arouses in those who are neither of the two);

3. is not exclusivist. Naked, semi-naked and fully bathing-costumed people live happily alongside each other in the Englische Garten and elsewhere. People strip off or remain clothed just as they please, often within the same group of sunbathers. Voyeurism (of which there is undoubtedly some) or the possibility of sexual arousal – two of the great anxieties which led to the strict rules in the institutionalisation of the Naturist movements – do not come

into play here. Or at least they do not create sufficient discomfort to the unclothed to change their practice nor do they cause rejection of those people who do not wish to strip.

What I would like to argue is that these cultural constructions of the naked body are not isolated instances in the UK and Germany, but are constitutive of one of our most body-centred leisure activities: the visit to the sauna. I will therefore begin by describing some very typical layouts of saunas in both countries. But before I enter into a more detailed comparison, I need to add a proviso: I am not saying that everything to do with saunas – the different layouts, instructions, rules or advice for use, and the social behaviour, attitudes and preferences of sauna users – is entirely determined by sociocultural attitudes about the unclothed body. This would be naive and superficial. There are many other structural, administrative or financial reasons why there are such strong contrasts in the physical layout of the average sauna in Germany and the UK, but such external restraints cannot explain away what amounts, in my view, to a very different predisposition towards the activity of sauna-going. It is this difference which is reflected in, and confirmed by, the physical layout of the saunas in both countries.

Sauna signs and signifiers in the UK and Germany

Typical layouts

I will begin by offering you some photographs that exemplify these differences in very obvious ways: see Figure 9.1 pictures (a) and (b) for the layout of the changing-room lockers and toilet, pictures (c) and (d) for the shower and rest area of a sauna in Southern England, and picture (e) for a typical sauna arrangement in a leisure centre in Southern Germany.

To be fair, the first set of pictures was taken in a publicly financed leisure centre (in the South of England), whereas the second comes from a private leisure centre in Bavaria – though it may come as a surprise that the cost for attending the German leisure centre is only slightly higher than that of attending the English version, and no different at all for a family ticket for four. There are, of course, some places in the UK which resemble the latter luxurious arrangements, though these tend to be exorbitantly priced. In contrast, it would be hard to find the equivalent of the UK examples in Germany. However,

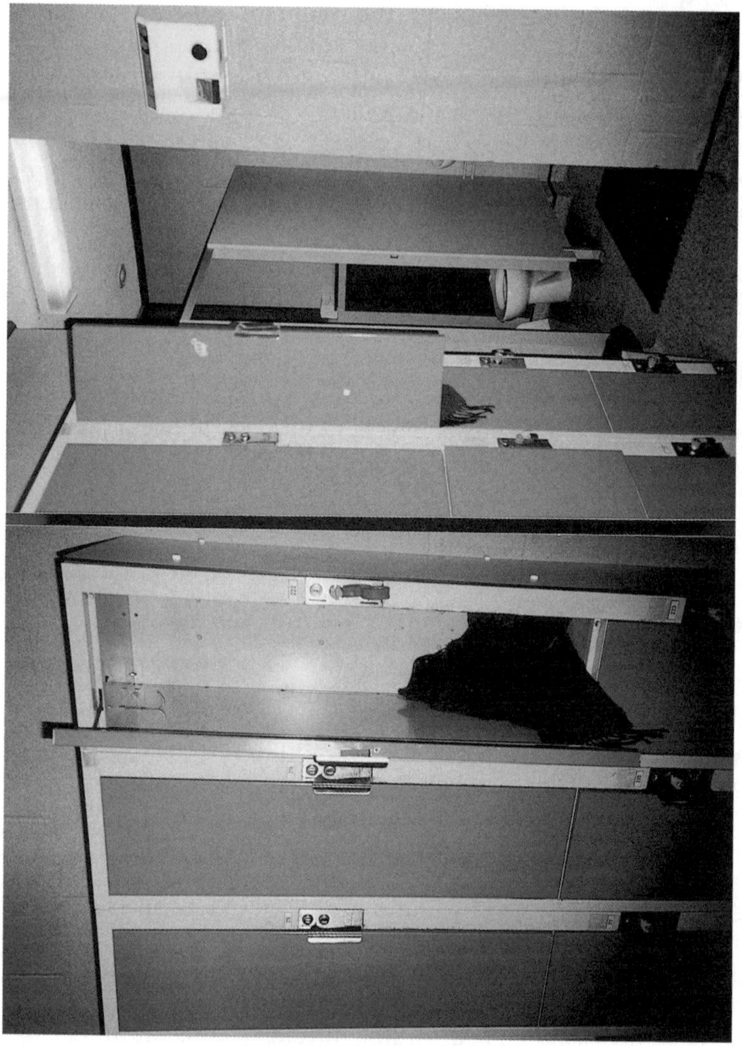

Figure 9.1 Picture (a) locker room   Picture (b) locker room with toilet

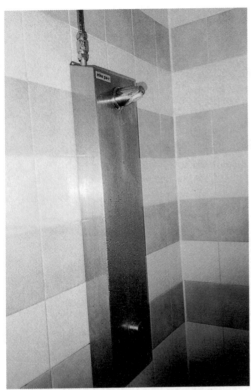

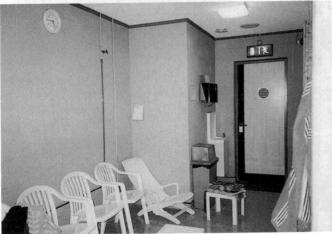

Figure 9.1 cont'd Picture (c) the shower(s) with fixed water temperature
Picture (d) the rest (or cooling-down) area with the door leading to the gym (the
door to the heated area is on the right behind the striped towel)

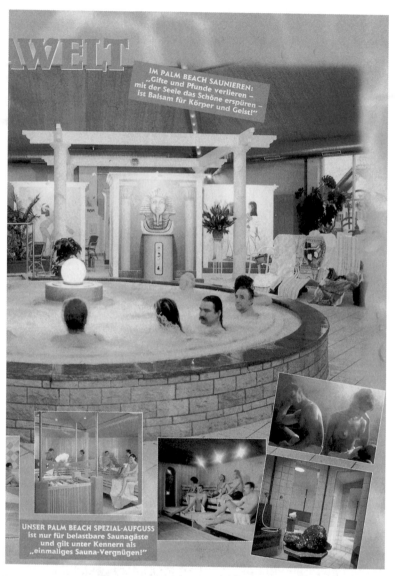

Figure 9.1 cont'd   Picture (e) (*top*) the Jacuzzi inside the rest area; (*below*) three shots taken inside the hot area and view of some of the shower facilities

my interest in this chapter is not in the saunas as such – though my examples should explain some of the culture-shock which German and British people experience in each others' saunas – but in the ways in which German or British discourses of and about saunas link in with particular constructions of the naked body.

British sauna provisions and messages

My argument goes as follows: more often than not, the British sauna experience sits uneasily at either end of a scale. At one end of this scale, the sauna is constructed as a sinful and sexually suspect, and hence by implication, a potentially unhealthy and dangerous site. Or, at the opposite end, it is constructed as a somewhat insignificant aspect of sport and fitness in general. This is often also architecturally marked: many saunas in public leisure centres are located next to the gym rather than the pool as they would be in their German equivalents, and more often than not come without any proper relaxation facilities, such as deck chairs for the cooling-off period, cooler and warmer resting rooms, or spaces for walking about in the cold. The provisions tend to be spartan as in the case shown in Figure 9.1, pictures 3c and d, where the rest area is restricted to a few plastic chairs in a small warm space immediately outside the hot part of the sauna, and next to the noise of the gym. Given the restricted space of this particular sauna there are nevertheless a number of signs displayed on its walls that give instructions and advice (see Figure 9.2, pictures a–d below).

These messages are somewhat contradictory: only the three signs in bold [red and] black lettering refer to the actual procedures and facilities available to the sauna-goer. The one that is headed 'Warning cold showers' (picture a) is particularly interesting.

Let us investigate this text in a little more detail:

WARNING COLD SHOWERS
DUE TO POPULAR DEMAND
THESE SHOWERS ARE NOW
SET ON COLD. HOT SHOWERS
ARE AVAILABLE
IN THE CHANGING AREAS.

The presupposition that is built into this text is that a proper shower is warm, not cold. Cold showers are something of which we need to be warned, as in line 1. Or, put differently, the unmarked idea of a British shower is warm, or even hot, even in a sauna, where health benefit and

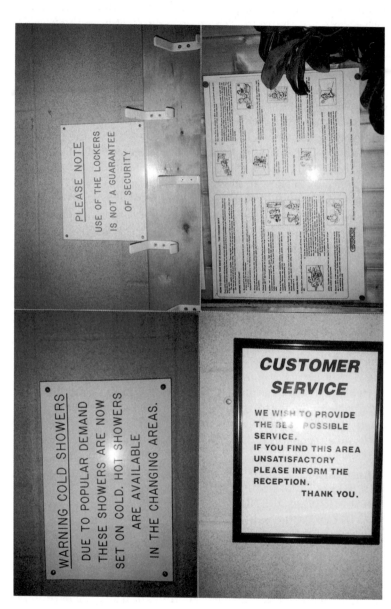

Figure 9.2 Pictures (a)–(d) contradictory messages

body pleasure for the visitors are supposed to derive from the rapid exchange between hot air and cold water, and the ensuing stimulation to their blood circulation. Here the coldness of the shower is such a marked idea, that a warning must be issued.

Lines 2–4 contain four propositions:

- first of all, we are told that there are cold showers, namely that is there is more than just one shower which yields cold water only. This could be misinterpreted since, as Figure 9.1(c) above shows, there is only one shower space, which does, however, contain two showers – one higher up and one lower down (see photograph);
- secondly, we must infer, that the temperature of these showers is unadjustable – they are either hot or cold;
- thirdly, and most importantly, we can infer that it was not the idea of the leisure-centre staff to put these on to cold but 'popular demand': it was the sauna-goers themselves who had asked for and were given cold showers in the sauna area;
- finally, we are reassured in lines 4–6 that there are indeed hot showers in the changing rooms (actually it is one hot shower in each of the male and female changing rooms, neither of which is adjustable either).

The other two notices in bold lettering (Figure 9.2(b)–(c)) also give helpful advice: they warn that the use of the lockers is not a guarantee of security – indeed it is not, as the broken lock of Figure 9.1 (a) shows – and they inform us that there is a customer service responsive to the customers' needs.

However, there is also a longer text which is not legible in the reproduction here because of its very small print (Figure 9.2 (d)). This text has comic-strip illustrations next to a text that explains exactly the 'do's and don'ts' for the sauna-goer, and stresses the health benefits that arise from proper behaviour. Apart from the tiny script, which renders this advice hardly legible, the advice itself cannot be followed in this sauna since it would be (1) illegal and (2) impossible to behave according to these instructions in this particular sauna. To isolate just a few of these:

- the comic-strip illustrations show naked people sitting on towels – but in this sauna it is not permitted to go without a swimming costume. Also, people do not usually bring towels to sit on, nor are they given any on entry;

- the comic strip and its text explain the importance of rest, and show a man happily stretched on a bed covered by a towel – a form of relaxation not really matching what is available in this sauna's one-and-only reclining plastic chair;
- it also tells you how good and healthy it is to take a swim in between your sauna sessions, but this activity is prevented by another sign on the exit/entrance to the sauna which informs you that, unless you are properly dry and dressed, you are not allowed to cross from that part of the building that houses the sauna (and the gym) to the other part of the leisure-centre that houses the pool, with the public entrance area in-between. In short, it is quite obvious that there is a hierarchy of instructions and advice in this sauna, with some signs signalling their importance by the topography of the lettering – capital letters in black or red bold script – whereas the other advisory text in small print and, illustrated through comic-strip figures can and indeed, must be disregarded.

This sauna is clearly an example of the post-gym work-out sauna on the puritan end of the scale. On the other end of the scale we do, of course, find a much more luxurious version in the UK as well, which is not positioned within ordinary everyday sport-and-leisure discourse. These are much more exclusivist in two important senses which often overlap: first, their hefty entry prices deter all but the financially unchallenged, and thus create a social form of exclusivity by default; secondly, many are perceived to be sexually marked even where they are not gender-exclusive. Neither attract the kind of mixed audience typical of the 'sporty' sauna in the UK or the vast majority of luxurious saunas in Germany. One instance of a socially exclusive sauna/pool, the Sanctuary in Covent Garden – which dwells on relaxation and luxury and resembles in its layout some of the German sauna spaces displayed in this chapter – is gender-exclusive in being restricted only to women. This could appear like an instance of the sexually exclusive since, given their women-only rule, the Sanctuary could be visited by lesbians and thus potentially attract the kind of reputation and anxiety that the (largely male and gay) Brighton beach arouses. However, I want to suggest that the framework of exclusivity (heightened by many cosmetic services on offer) created in the space of the Sanctuary addresses high-earning professional women, and their wish to be free from the male gaze, rather than invites single-sex opportunities for arousal or voyeurism. Hence its social exclusivity based on income and gender allows professional women to escape rather than embrace what might otherwise be constructed as a sexually marked space. By comparison, those expensive saunas that try to incorporate the relaxed, leisurely and atmospheric without wanting to deter a mixed-gender clientele can find themselves in a dilemma, precisely because of the suspicion of sexual innuendo that easily attaches itself to such spaces of leisure. One Brighton sauna, for example, housed in a five-storey town house is a particularly obvious instance of this phenomenon: rich on atmospheric signs of relaxation and pleasure with grottoes and small pools,subdued lights, a bar and a rest area under a glass roof with a balcony, it feels obliged to make a rule that states that on Saturday and Sunday after 5pm, only mixed-gender couples are allowed to visit. In addition, it also gives such couples at all times a huge price reduction. Like the institutionalised nudist spaces referred to above, this Brighton sauna has behavioural norms that make nakedness obligatory – except for towels which are permitted to be 'worn' – in all the spaces including those of the bar and the rest area: a sarong, just to add some anecdotal evidence, was already interpreted as 'dress' and hence prohibited. This rule-enforcement echoes the anxieties of other obligatory nudist spaces implying that anyone clothed amongst the otherwise unclothed must have suspect motives.

Texts of German 'saunalands'

Let us now, by contrast, examine some of the discourses to be found in and about German saunas. I have selected extracts from two pamphlets from saunas in Upper Frankonia- one is near Nürnberg, another is near a smaller town close by (Herzogenaurach) – and add to these some photographs of my own. These pamphlets, of course, are a different type of text from the signs and posters that I analysed in the section above. However, many of the 'texts' that appear in the pamphlet are also on display on the walls of the saunas that they advertise. In any case, I am using these texts as indicative of the ways in which the experience of sauna-going is being constructed by a whole range of different texts. They are typical instances for a collection of other, similar material on which I could have drawn. The pamphlets in question are displayed at the entrance or in the eating areas of the leisure-centres they refer to, both of which are privately run facilities but with entry prices which do not differ much from their public counterparts. Both have exotic names: 'Atlantis' is the name of one, and 'Palm Beach' is the name of the other. However, in spite of this stress on the exotic in the names, what I want to show is that in these texts, and indeed in the layout and provisions offered by the centres, the sauna experience is part of a much more all-embracing range of activities. Exoticism is only one of a whole range of different and potentially contradictory discourses, sitting alongside those of tradition and mysticism but also of sport, health, relaxation, leisure and family fun. In this respect, there is a sharp difference not only from the English saunaland, but also to the other more closely related tradition of the Finnish sauna.

Sauna and cultural identity: the case of the Finnish Sauna

A brief excursion into the significance of the Finnish sauna will make this clear. To my knowledge and with the notable exception of Norden (1987), the Finnish sauna is the only tradition that has so far found its entry into the academic literature. It is said to be so implicated with Finnish ethnicity that it is placed in the tradition of magic healing (Achte, 1997) psychiatric healing (Sorri, 1988), and mentioned alongside other (high) culture icons of Finnishness such as the composer Sibelius (Stoller, 1996). It is always described and narrativised as essentially and quintessentially Finnish. Below is an extract from one of several web pages that provide elegaic accounts of the sauna experience and link this with every aspect of being Finnish:

> The origins of the Northern sauna are lost in the mists of prehistory, but the word is Finnish (correctly pronounced sow-na, rather than saw-na) and, if the Finns were not the creators of the practice, it has been far more important to their recorded culture than to that of any other European people. The Kalevala, Finland's national epic (which contains much religious and traditional material) includes several sequences describing the importance of sauna as a social activity, a place for giving birth, and simply one of the finest pleasures of home.
>
> (http://www.birchlake.com/CoolPages/SaunaDesc.html)

According to this literature, the Finnish sauna to the Finns is so inextricably part of their traditions, their mythologies and deepest cultural roots, that going to the sauna – whether this is at home or as an expat Finn anywhere in the world (Ladenheim, 1998; Lipson *et al.*, 1984) – is an acting out and 'daily confirmation' (Billig, 1995) of being Finnish. To the 'imagined community' (Anderson, 1983), of the Finns, sauna-going is one of its key confirmatory elements of cultural identity. (For a critical discussion of Finnish myth-construction around their sauna, see Edelsward, 1991).

By contrast, the mixture of discourses that we find in the German pamphlets about saunas does not in any way attempt to construct a particularly German identity, but involves much more superficial, though highly hedonistic, pick-and-mix notions of health, pleasure and leisure for the self, the group or the family. Other cultural traditions are imported as postmodern quotations, creating a bricolage of eclectic cultural reference points: mystical, exotic, sensuous. All of this is brought under some kind of umbrella by the old Roman philosophical ideal of 'means sana in corpore sano'. This unifying notion of a healthy body, a healthy mind and a healthy soul is rhetorically put to work, underpinning the different references and dissolving any possible contradictions arising from them.

Pick-and-mix discourses of the German sauna

Text 1: the Atlantis

I will now give some examples from the pamphlets in question, with my translations staying as close to the German original as possible, even where this may produce somewhat inelegant English.

These two facing pages construct two very different discourses. Page 2 of the leaflet (Figure 9.3(a)) mainly emphasises Bavarian traditional aspects, whereas page 3 (Figure 9.3(b)) combines mysticism and exoticism with relaxation. The Bavarian reference needs some comment. Although the Atlantis is in the federal state of Bavaria, its local region is Upper Frankonia, which has different traditions and a very different dialect from Upper-Bavaria. Nevertheless, text and pictures draw on a 'native tradition' of Bavarian architecture and language. On page 2, and below the photograph of what looks like a typical Southern-Bavarian farmhouse from the outside, we find a drawing of the inside of this farmhouse converted to a sauna. The text underlines this Bavarian tradition in several ways:

- traditional building material (wood) and its age (having been passed on from one generation to the next):

Top section: column 1
For two hundred years, this beautiful house built entirely from wood, was handed down from one generation to the next
(Zweihundert Jahre lang wurde das wunderschöne, ganz aus Holz errichtete bayerische Bauernhaus von Generation zu Generation vererbt);

192

Zweihundert Jahre lang wurde das wunderschöne, ganz aus Holz errichtete bayerische Bauernhaus von Generation zu Generation vererbt. Dann wollte niemand mehr in dem „alten Graffl" wohnen: zu unmodern, kein Komfort, alter Steinofen statt moderner Zentralheizung. Dem rustikalen Holzhaus, Fachleute nennen es ein „Stockhaus", drohte zunächst das gleiche Schicksal wie vielen anderen, nämlich einfach verfeuert zu werden. Aber das Haus konnte gerettet werden. Es wird zu einer Sauna im original bayerischen Bauernhaus umgebaut. Nun warten die alten Bohlen und Balken fein säuberlich numeriert und konserviert auf ein neues Leben.

Eine wirklich „heiße" Nachricht:

Atlantis bekommt neue Aufgußsauna

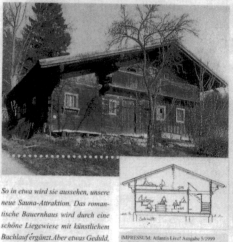

So in etwa wird sie aussehen, unsere neue Sauna-Attraktion. Das romantische Bauernhaus wird durch eine schöne Liegewiese mit künstlichem Bachlauf ergänzt. Aber etwas Geduld, bitte, denn die Einweihung feiern wir mit Ihnen im Herbst.

IMPRESSUM: Atlantis Live! Ausgabe 5/1999
V.i.S.d.P.: Idee und Konzept: Wolfgang Schneider
Realisierung: con pro GmbH, Naunhof
Fotografen: Udo Dreier, Klaus Batz, Wolfgang Roeske, Atlantis-Bildarchiv

Unsere Saunagäste dürfen sich auf diese neue Attraktion freuen. Ganz aus Holz und richtig urig wird die neue Aufgußsauna werden. Ab Herbst wird es in ihr jedenfalls ziemlich heiß hergehen.

Für die rustikale Sauna mit Platz für mindestens 40 Personen wird der Atlantis-Saunagarten entsprechend erweitert. Unsere Gäste sollen dadurch ein noch besseres Angebot bekommen. Das ist auch ein kleiner Dank für den tollen Zuspruch, den unsere Atlantis-Sauna seit ihrer Eröffnung erfahren hat. Weil es bei den heißbegehrten Aufgüssen inzwischen wegen des großen Zuspruchs manchmal etwas eng wird, soll die neue Sauna Abhilfe schaffen. Damit Sie das Vergnügen noch mehr genießen können! In der unverwechselbaren Atmosphäre eines alten Bauernhofs. Auf geht's Buam und Madeln, pack'mers an!

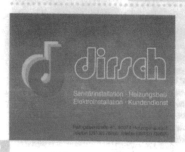
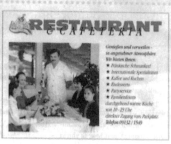
Figure 9.3   The Atlantis   (a) Lefthand page (2) of leaflet

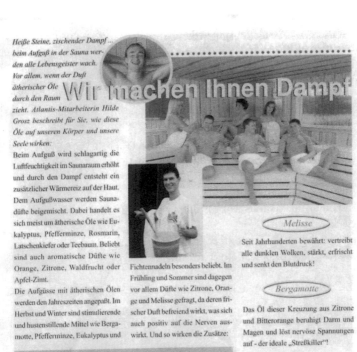

Heiße Steine, zischender Dampf ... beim Aufguß in der Sauna werden alle Lebensgeister wach. Vor allem, wenn der Duft ätherischer Öle durch den Raum zieht. Atlantis-Mitarbeiterin Hilde Grosz beschreibt für Sie, wie diese Öle auf unseren Körper und unsere Seele wirken:

Wir machen Ihnen Dampf

Beim Aufguß wird schlagartig die Luftfeuchtigkeit im Saunaraum erhöht und durch den Dampf entsteht ein zusätzlicher Wärmereiz auf der Haut. Dem Aufgußwasser werden Saunadüfte beigemischt. Dabei handelt es sich meist um ätherische Öle wie Eukalyptus, Pfefferminze, Rosmarin, Latschenkiefer oder Teebaum. Beliebt sind auch aromatische Düfte wie Orange, Zitrone, Waldfrucht oder Apfel-Zimt.

Die Aufgüsse mit ätherischen Ölen werden den Jahreszeiten angepaßt. Im Herbst und Winter sind stimulierende und hustenstillende Mittel wie Bergamotte, Pfefferminze, Eukalyptus und Fichtennadeln besonders beliebt. Im Frühling und Sommer sind dagegen vor allem Düfte wie Zitrone, Orange und Melisse gefragt, da deren frischer Duft befreiend wirkt, was sich auch positiv auf die Nerven auswirkt. Und so wirken die Zusätze:

Melisse

Seit Jahrhunderten bewährt: vertreibt alle dunklen Wolken, stärkt, erfrischt und senkt den Blutdruck!

Bergamotte

Das Öl dieser Kreuzung aus Zitrone und Bitterorange beruhigt Darm und Magen und löst nervöse Spannungen auf - der ideale „Streßkiller"!

Minze

Ein ziemlich „cooler" Duft, denn das Öl der Pfefferminze reizt die kälteempfindlichen Nerven. Es ist schmerzstillend, krampflösend und sorgt für einen klaren Kopf.

Teebaum

Der „Tea tree" hat mit den Pflanzen, aus denen der grüne und schwarze Tee gewonnen wird, nichts zu tun. Sein kostbares Öl bringt Bakterien und Viren zur Strecke. Und der ungewöhnliche Duft schafft, zugegeben, auch so manchen geruchsempfindlichen Saunafan!

„Kraulbrustrücken"

„Schwimmen ist gesund" - eine Alltagsweisheit. Aber wußten Sie auch, warum Schwimmen tatsächlich eine der gesündesten Sportarten ist? Es ist eine Ausdauersportart, bei der alle Muskelgruppen effektiv trainiert werden können. Durch den Auftrieb werden die Gelenke geschont und die Haltung verbessert. Und durch den Kältereiz und die Belastung läuft unser „Motor" auf Hochtouren. Die Atmung wird verbessert, der Stoffwechsel gesteigert und die Durchblutung gefördert. Unsere körpereigene Zentralheizung wird mal so richtig „durchgepustet". Wichtig: vorher aufwärmen und die Muskeln dehnen, gleich nach dem Schwimmen ins Trockene und Warme. Und beim Training nichts übertreiben!

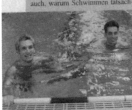

Figure 9.3   The Atlantis   (b) righthand page (3) of leaflet

- dialectal phrasing:
  'Urig' – this word is impossible to translate but its connotations are traditional Bavarian style and atmosphere:

Middle section: column 3
Made entirely out of wood and really 'urig'
(Ganz aus Holz und richtig urig . . .);

'Buam and Madeln, pack' mers an'. Also Upper-Bavarian rather than local Frankonian dialect for 'boys and girls':

Bottom section: column 3
In the unmistakable athmosphere of an old farmhouse. 'Let's have a go, boys and girls'
(In der unverwechselbaren Atmosphäre eines alten Bauernhofs. Auf geht's Buam und Madeln, pack' mers an)

- the risk to its survival as a farmhouse in the modern world (column 2);
- the rescue of the house by its conversion into the Atlantis sauna (column 3):

But the house was saved. It is now being converted into a sauna inside the original Bavarian farmhouse.

(Aber das Haus konnte gerettet werden. Es wird zu einer Sauna im original bayerischen Bauernhaus umgebaut).

Page 3 of the leaflet (Figure 9.3 (b)), by contrast plays on exoticism, mysticism, relaxation, health and fun.
  Below are some examples:

- Relaxation and pleasure:
  The photograph shows a group of smiling sauna-goers, coyly displayed as they sit in the sauna wrapped in towels.

- Mysticism and exoticism:
  Hot stones, fizzing steam . . . through the 'Aufguß' {1} in the sauna all energies are awakened (literally: all life-spirits, but the expression 'Lebensgeister' in German has become idiomatic-colloquial). Especially when the scent of ethereal oils drifts through the room.

Atlantis employee Hilde Grosz describes how these oils affect our body and our soul.

Heiße Steine, zischender Dampf . . . beim Aufguß in der Sauna werden alle Lebensgeister wach. Vor allem, wenn der Duft ätherischer Öle durch den Raum zieht. Atlantis-Mitarbeiterin Hilde Grosz beschreibt für Sie, wie diese Öle auf unseren Körper und unsere Seele wirken.

- Health:
The rest of the page is devoted to a detailed account of the health benefits accruing from the sauna, using a mixture of colloquial and medical language:

> . . . through the steam there develops an additional heat stimulus on the skin (middle section, column 1)
> . . . durch den Dampf entsteht ein zusätzlicher Wärmereiz auf der Haut

> . . . a stimulating and cough-reducing herb (bottom Section column 1)
> . . . stimulierende und hustenstillende Mittel

> Balm-mint . . . strengthens, refreshes and lowers blood-pressure (column 3)
> Melisse . . . stärkt, erfrischt und senkt den Blutdruck

> Bergamot . . . calms intestines and stomach
> Bergamotte . . . beruhigt Darm und Magen

> Mint: pain-reducing, cramp-dissolving, gives you a clear head
> Minze . . . schmerzstillend, krampflösend und sorgt für einen kearen Kopf

> tea-tree . . . kills off bacteria and viruses
> Teebaum . . . bringt Bakterien und Viren zur Strecke.

But apart from these more straightforward and detailed health benefits, here we also get more exotic and mystical combinations:

> ethereal oils such as eucalypthus, peppermint, rosemary (column 1)
> aromatic scents such as orange, lemon . . .
> ätherische Öle wie Eukalyptus, Pfefferminze, Rosmarin . . .
> aromatische Düfte wie Orange, Zitrone . . .

and combination of body and 'soul' effects:

> . . . since their fresh scent has a liberating effect, which positively affects your nerves (column 2)
> . . . da deren frischer Duft befreiend wirkt, was sich auch positiv auf die Nerven auswirkt

> Balm-mint . . . disperses all dark clouds (column 3)
> Bergamot . . . dissolves nervous tensions . . . the ideal stress-killer
> Mint . . . stimulates those nerves that are sensitive to cold weather.

> Melisse . . . vertreibt alle dunklen Wolken
> Bergamotte . . . löst nervöse Spanungen auf- de rideale Streßkiller
> Minze . . . reizt die kälteempfindlichen Nerven.

The most interesting aspect of this text is its total pick-and-mix discourse. The sauna not only represents any number of desirable aspects of leisured life by the images we are shown and by the promised effects; it also allows any number of in-groups to cohabit – the youngish people on the picture, the traditional boys and girls, the health-conscious and the modern mystic. The language echoes that by drawing on different styles and registers side by side. The health discourse is largely realised through generalised descriptive factual terms, with no addressee or no one person grammaticalised as a direct beneficiary. It is the oil or the scent acting directly on the nerves or the stomach or the blood pressure. In that sense the language is similar to that found on leaflets in boxes of tablets which also itemise the effects the medicament is intended to have on specific parts of the body. Or it is a passive construction of factuality (Beim Aufguß wird . . . die Luftfeuchtigkeit im Saunaraum erhöht – the humidity in the sauna room is increased as a result of an Aufguß, column 1). But these impersonalised constructions are interwoven with the 'you' and 'us' discourse, where the 'du' – group of the 'Buam and Madel' (the boys and girls), and the 'Sie' group of 'you our sauna-guests' again live happily side by side. There is some play with the metaphoric use of 'hot' – heiß, since 'heiß' in German is often used as a colloquial expression meaning something similar to the English use of 'cool' as 'great' or 'super' (the latter is also used in German but in its borrowed English form), or just as an intensifier, and without any obvious sexual insinuations:

> eine wirklich heiße Nachricht = a really super bit of news
> heißbegehrte Aufguß- the hotly (or much) desired Aufguß

In fact, I would argue that even where the idiom normally would arouse sexual innuendo, as in 'ab Herbst wird es in ihr jedenfalls *ziemlich heiß hergehen*' (from the autumn it will be pretty steamy in here), the sexual connotation of the expression is only there as a pun on the factual literal heat of the sauna. If I am right, and I have to accept that there may be other readings of this, then this is a really interesting counter-example to the anxiety of the Brighton sauna I mentioned before: this German sauna can afford to create a wordplay with a pun on a possible, if slight, sexual innuendo. Nothing, it seems, could be further from anyone's mind in this context. The wordplay around notions of 'hot' rather fits in with other metaphoric puns on the notion of heat and steam, as in the header 'wir machen ihnen Dampf', literally 'we make you steam' which metaphorically means something like 'we get you going' or 'we speed you up'.

Text 2: the Palm Beach

My second German example comes from the Palm Beach pamphlet. Here, the pick-and-mix sauna discourses are developed in an even more elaborated fashion. The front page of the pamphlet (see Figure 9.4) sets the agenda for the booklet as a whole by interspersing photos with logos and with text captions.

The title caption, 'Spa and leisure pool', names health and leisure. The picture underneath on the left has the logo with the name, the metonymic palm tree, the sun and the sea wave, a combination for which the industrial suburb of Stein near Nuremberg is not exactly known. On the right, also in logo form, a crystal: one of the main themes of mystical purity on which this sauna draws heavily. In the middle, two photos, which index the types of leisure on offer, show a man and a woman looking away from one another glowing in the sauna, obviously naked but coyly photographed; on the other the same man and woman now holding one another and laughing in the water.

The caption in the middle gives the location ('In Stein bei Nürnberg' written in the form of a wave), above a straight caption which reads: Erholung für Körper, Geist und Seele (Relaxation for body, mind and soul).

The photo below that stresses family fun by showing the wave pool with the inflatable octopus and lots of young people. This is framed by the text on the left which names the activities in the leisure-centre: 'Schwimmen, Saunieren, Kneippen, Rutschen' (swimming, saunaing, 'Kneippen' (2), sliding) and on the right by naming the benefit which these activities produce: 'Wohlfühlen, Entspannen, Genießen, Relaxen' (feeling good, taking away tension, enjoying, relaxing).

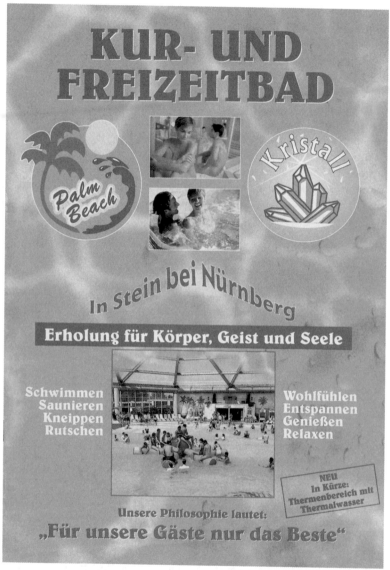

Figure 9.4 **The Palm Beach** Front page

And finally at the bottom we find the 'philosophy' rhyme: 'Für unsere Gäste nur das Beste' (only the best for our guests).

Inside, the sixteen-page thick glossy brochure is packed full of information in text and image, of which the following are the most significant for the sauna aspect of the leisure-centre:

- A list of provisions. Much emphasis is placed on the variety of provisions to cover every possible form and taste for taking saunas. There are three sauna sections covered on three double-sided pages: the 'Sauna world', the 'Sauna village', and the Turkish/Osmanic sauna: Saunawelt: comprises the 'Sauna park' with a large sauna for special 'Aufguß', a smaller Finnish Sauna, three steam temples (Dampftempel); a bio-sauna Saunadorf. The all-year-round outdoors Sauna village comprises several houses, (reachable in winter by running across the snowy meadow and crossing icy little bridges) which contain the gem sauna (Edelsteinsauna,) the hay sauna (Heusauna,) the lemon-aroma sauna (Zitronen-Aromasauna), two Finnish saunas, a special 'Herrensauna' (gentlemen's sauna), and a Kindersauna (children's sauna) The Turkish-Osmanic area of the leisure-centre boasts a 'marble sweat-stone' and a 'fountain of youth'.
- Body, mind and soul experiences: relaxation, purification and mysticism. As important as the range of activities is the range of different body-and-soul experiences they engender, which are couched in a mixture of descriptive, rhapsodic, metaphoric and poetic styles.

The indoor area of the Saunawelt (Sauna world) draws more on the mixture of exotic (Roman, Finnish and Egyptian) cultures, whereas the outside area, the Saunadorf (sauna village), with its individual small Bavarian-style huts, again draws on Upper-Bavarian traditions. Here a whole set of small sauna huts are built as a miniature version of original houses in Oberammergau, a village made famous by its annual Passion plays- complete with a copy of the highest German mountain (Zugspitze) and imitation waterfall. As in the case of the Atlantis, a Southern-Bavarian tradition is brought in instead of the more local Frankonian one:

With a waterfall at the 'Zugspitze' (the highest German mountain), a mountain brook, ponds, the market square with a linden tree, a wonderful beer garden and many rest areas- here you find a sauna village extraordinarily and amiably designed.
Mit Wasserfall an der Zugspitze, Gebirgsbach, Teichen, dem Marktplatz mit Dorflinde, einem herrlichen Biergarten und vielen

Ruhezonen, finden Sie hier ein Saunadorf so außergewöhnlich wie liebevoll gestaltet.

Examples from the 'Saunawelt':

• Descriptive:

To do sauna is relaxing for body, mind and soul
Saunieren ist Relaxen für Körper, Geist und Seele

• Rhapsodic:

According to Hildegard von Bingen (identified later in the pamphlet as 'eine Weltheilige', a world saint), mountain crystals have a purifying effect for body, mind and soul. But even if you don't wish to believe this, you will not be able to withdraw from the fascination of its special light.
Bergkristalle haben nach Hildegard von Bingen eine reinigende Wirkung auf Körper, Geist und Seele. Aber selbst wenn Sie nicht daran glauben mögen, werden Sie sich der Faszination dieses besonderen Lichtes nicht entziehen können.

• Therapeutic:

integrated colour and light therapy
integrierte Farb- und Lichttherapie

• Poetic:

To do sauna in the Palm Beach
to shed poison and pounds
to reach beauty with your soul
is balm for body and spirit.

Im Palm Beach saunieren,
Gifte und Pfunde verlieren-
mit der Seele das Schöne erspüren
ist Balsam für Körper und Geist.

In the Saunadorf, the main focus is on the health benefit of the sauna (the hay sauna, for example, is said to have direct and beneficial effects on health). As with the Atlantis, the activities associated with the German spa tradition and their benefit for one's physical health are invoked through factual descriptive language for the exchanges between hot and cold water, and medical vocabulary for the body itself. Kneippen comprises a whole gamut of such activities: hot-cold foot-baths (Wechselfußbäder), whole-body showering (Ganzkörperduschen), cold-water showers (Kaltwassergüssen), foot-reflex massage (Fußreflexmassage) through treading water on pebbles (Wassertreten auf Kieselsteinen), all of which act beneficially on the 'metabolism' (Stoffwechsel) and on the 'blood circulation' (Kreislauf) of those who engage in them.

This descriptive health-related discourse then culminates in a holistic celebration of the general quality of life:

> For a long time 'doing sauna' has not been merely sweating the body. Sauna is today a form of quality of life, relaxation for the body, mind/spirit and soul.
> Saunieren ist schon lange nicht mehr nur 'Schwitzen des Körpers', Saunieren ist heute eine Art Lebensqualität, Erholung für Körper, Geist und Seele geworden.

In the Turkish-Osmanic area, the notion of 'kneippen' is combined with orientally inspired ideas about the body and the soul. Here the mystical and exotic is at its most pronounced.

> 'Kneippen': an ideal fountain of youth
> Kneippen: Ein idealer Jungbrunnen (mythical)

> The purpose of indulging in Hamam was physical and spiritual purification, the shedding of thoughts from ordinary existence, the relaxation of joints and muscles and thus also mental relaxation.
> Ziel des Hamam – Genusses was die körperliche und geistige Reinigung, das Abstreifen der Alltagsgedanken, das Lockern der Gelenke und Muskeln und damit auch geistge Erholung.

> As long as 800 years ago, long before there were washing facilities in the European regal and ducal homes, the Osmanic rulers together with their teachers of Islam developed a high culture of bathing which culminated in the so-called Hamam.
> (Schon vor 800 Jahren, lange bevor an den Europäischen Fürsten- und Königshäusern Waschgelegenheiten eingerichtet wurden,

entwickelten die osmanischen Herrscher zusammen mit ihren islamischen Religionslehrern eine hochstehende Badekultur, die im sogenannten Hamam ihre Krönung fand.)

Although these texts show that the different zones of the sauna have their prevalent discourses which link them with particular aesthetic, geographical or cultural traditions, there is also – just as in the Atlantis – a great deal of mixing even within the same space.

In both the 'Saunawelt' and the Turkish-Osmanic area, for example, the exotic discourses quoted above are complemented by purely factual, descriptive accounts of the facilities and decorations on offer, as follows:

- The mountain crystals:

  The sauna park is lit by 240 Brazilian mountain crystals on the ceiling and one crystal ball in the middle of its large hot-whirlpool.
  der Saunapark wird durch 240 brasilianische Bergkristalle an der Decke und einer Kristallkugel in der Mitte des großen Hot-Whirlpool beleuchtet.

- Turkish marble:

  As in earlier times, original Turkish marble was used in its design from mines near to the Black Sea and adapted to the original Osmanic style. There are 240 stars in the cupola, lit by glass fibre.
  Bei der Gestaltung wurde wie auch früher schon original türkischer Marmor aus Steinbrüchen nahe des Schwarzen Meeres verwendet und auf den original osmanischen Stil abgestellt. In der Kuppel sind 240 Sterne, die durch Glasfaser beleuchtet werden, angebracht.

- The murals:

  Artistically high-quality wall paintings from the different epochs of bathing cultures.
  Künstlerische hochwertig gestaltete Wandmalereien aus den verschiedenen Badeepochen.

For English readers, texts such as these invite camp readings. However, in the context of these German saunas, this would be a mistake. The exoticism referred to above, which ranges on the absurd, is happily interwoven with the discourses of straightforward leisure and fun, regional-home traditions, friends and family:

- Saunawelt:

  'gemütliche' Sauna bar with open fire, amidst lovely people
  gemütliche Saunabar am Kaminfeuer, inmitten netter Leute

- Saunadorf:

  In the sauna village you can also find a children's playground (a creche) with playing facilities and a children's sauna at 40 centigrade for the little ones.
  Im Saunadorf sind auch ein Kinderhort mit Spielgeräten und eine Kindersauna mit 40 Grad Temperatur für die Kleinen zu finden.

Conclusion

I have argued that discourses of and about the sauna carry powerful messages about the body and bodies. These provide intriguing instances for cross-cultural differences between Britain and Germany. I think it is no exaggeration to say that the range of discourses which I have discussed, as well as some of the behaviour (running across icy meadows in the nude and standing underneath a fake waterfall at freezing temperatures), may come across to a British audience as over the top and potentially camp. Similarly, a German sauna-goer, confronted by English notices that warn of cold showers without even producing more than a tepid trickle, and people in bathing costumes sitting on wet sweaty wood without even the smallest towel underneath, would treat this as deeply offensive, and dangerous to life and limb.

On the other hand, the more extravagant mystic and exotic rhetorics of the German 'saunaland' pass largely unnoticed inside the naturalised setting of a German sauna-cum-leisure centre. After all, people do not actually read these pamphlets in any attentive way. Any further expansion of sauna provisions through exoticised spaces is simply enjoyed as yet another comfortable addition to leisure and relaxation rather than a journey into the soul. Clearly the German sauna appeals to a more general cultural predisposition where people enjoy relaxing in the nude without much further ado. There is a general conviction that being nude in a sauna is appropriate, healthy and fun – and you don't need a spare bathing costume when you go back to the swimming area. Hence the pamphlets with their fake traditions and insistence on exotic cultural histories make unintentionally funny reading.

By contrast, pieces in the British press, such as those selected from the *Guardian* – with headlines such as 'Tesco lays bare plans for shoppers' nudist night' (11 January 99) to TV reviews 'Jim Shelley refuses to let it all hang out' (21 November 98) or 'As naked as nature never intended' (10 October 86, see also extract below) – all play on the double take of the body as something that really and truly ought to be covered up. Such pieces are as intentionally funny as some of the discourses about nudity in the German sauna unintentionally verge on the absurd.

A quote from Judy Gahagan about the naked Germans in the Englische Garten highlights this clash of cultures in an amusingly ironic way:

> The fall was supposed to have brought us knowledge, sin and a sense of guilt and shame. In a word, everything that makes sex worthwhile. In a word everything that makes us different from animals. It is human to have an irrational sense of modesty, to wish to hide things about oneself, to feel a bit unworthy. And here were thousands of happy brown Germans without a shadow of Angst, immodestly and freely enjoying God's gifts without a stitch on. 'You don't know what you're missing', I wanted to shout.
>
> (*Guardian*, October 1986, p. 10)

Notes

1. Aufguβ is a word for which I cannot think of an English equivalent. It is the liquid consisting of water and drops of oil that is thrown on to the sauna-stove to create steam and release the scent, and with it the implied healing or relaxing powers of the oils. Once the 'Aufguβ' has been delivered it is not accepted behaviour to leave the sauna before at least five minutes have elapsed so as not to let the precious scents escape.
2. Kneipen refers to a form of spa cure based on Sebastian Kneipp's Wasserheilkunde of 1860, propagating rapid exchanges of hot and cold water for parts or the whole of the body. Kneipp, born in Bavaria and a church minister, was a medical layman whose work is today accepted by mainstream medicine for his holistic approach, with his therapies widely practised in German spas, and in particular in the spa town of Bad Wörishofen, the place where he worked and died.

References

Achte, K. (1997) 'Die alte finnische Mythologie von der Psychiatrie her betrachtet'. *Nervenheilkunde* 16: 291–3.

Anderson, B. (1983) *Imagined Communities*. London: Verso

Billig, M. (1995) *Banal Nationalism*. London: Sage.

Brown, R. and Gilman, Albert (1960/1972) 'The Pronouns of Power and Solidarity'. In P.P. Giglioli (ed.) (1972) *Language in Social Context*. Harmondsworth: Penguin, 252–82.

Edelsward, L.M. (1991) *Sauna as Symbol: Society and Culture in Finland*. Bern and New York: Peter Lang.

Ladenheim, M. (1998) *The Sauna in Central New York*. Dewitt: Historical Society.

Lipson, A.H., Webster, W.S. and Edwards, M.J. (1984) 'Attitudes to Sauna of Finnish expatriats and Australian Adults. *Teratology* 30:1.

Norden, Gilbert (1987) *Saunakultur in Österreich. Zur Soziologie der Sauna und des Saunabesuchs*. Wien: Böhlau.

Sorri, P. (1988) 'The Sauna and Sauna-bathing Habits: a Psychoanalytical Point of View'. *The Annals of Clinical Research* 20: 236–39.

Stoller, E.P. (1996) 'Sauna, Sisu and Sibelius: Ethnic Identity Among Finnish Americans'. *Sociological Quarterly*, 37 (1): 145–75.

Sauna web page:
www.birchlake.com/CoolPages/SaunaDesc.html

Part 3

The Body, Pathology and Constructions of Selfhood

10
Processes of Refiguration: Shifting Identities in Cancer Narratives

Richard Gwyn

In a prose poem by Robert Hass entitled 'A story about the body' (1989: 32), a young composer at an artists' colony becomes infatuated with a Japanese woman painter considerably older than himself. He considers the way she moves her body, the ways in which she uses her hands, and her 'amused and considered answers to his questions'. One evening, returning from a concert together, she tells him that she knows he is attracted to her, as she is to him, but if they are to make love he must know, she says, that she has had a double mastectomy. He appears not to understand, so she says: 'I've lost both my breasts.' The 'radiance' which the young composer 'had carried around in his belly and chest cavity withered very quickly', and he forces himself to face the woman and say: 'I'm sorry. I don't think I could.' The text continues:

> He walked back to his own cabin through the pines, and in the morning he found a small blue bowl on the porch outside his door. It looked to be full of rose petals, but he found when he picked it up that the rose petals were on top; the rest of the bowl – she must have swept them from the corners of her studio – was full of dead bees.

Here the predictability of the young man's assumptions about another's body is contrasted with the unpredictability of the real world, and the poem serves, in part at least, as a gendered and ironic statement on the nature of expectation and desire. Thus, when the young man finds the blue bowl on his porch the following morning, the allegorical arrangement of dead bees hidden by the rose petals makes explicit to him the embodied nature of his expectation, and reminds us, the readers, that an idealised and presumed body might be merely obscuring something as strange, as 'other', and as aesthetically unacceptable as 'a sweeping of dead bees'.

The threat to a constituted identity which cancer brings with it is the main topic of this chapter, and it is just such challenges to the ortho-doxy of expectation that cancer patients describe encountering again and again. There are a variety of channels through which these experi-ences are related, but they can be found embedded within extended oral or written narratives, for instance in the field of 'life writing', an autobiographical genre which has emerged in recent years (see, for example, Josselson and Lieblich, 1996), or else as recorded data col-lected by sociologists of health and illness. Television, a medium obsessed with tales of sickness and resistance to it, provides a vehicle for many such accounts and there is currently being shown, at the time of writing, a BBC television series dedicated specifically to the life narratives of people with cancer. Indeed, recent years have seen a glut of 'celebrity' accounts of illness experience, written by movie stars, authors, journalists and even social scientists.

In the pages that follow I will approach three interrelated objectives. First, I will examine the ways in which the concept of refiguration is explored in two recent accounts of cancer experience by a well-known journalist and a feminist novelist. Secondly, I will bring together salient themes within these and other accounts, and consider them within the general rubric of the mythic 'journey' described by Frank (1995); and thirdly, I will examine how we might do social science in the ambiguous zone between autobiographical writing and reflexive ethnography.

I would then, in the first instance, like to consider two 'popular' examples of texts upon the self, *A Season in Hell*, by the novelist and literary critic Marilyn French, and *C: Because Cowards Get Cancer Too*, by the late John Diamond, which also served as the basis for a TV film. I want to concentrate on the ways in which identity is discussed in these works, and especially the way in which identity is embodied, quite literally, in the physical changes incurred by the writers' experi-ences of cancer. The storyteller's body finds voice in these and similar accounts, and through these voicings and other tales of refiguration I hope to show that there are mutable and *owned* modes of narrativisa-tion that can impact on the broader aims of social science, helping to deconstruct the notion of an implacable and measurable science of researcher-led, non-participant observation; or the ideal of a profes-sionally detached 'data gathering' (cf. Geertz, 1988; Paget, 1995).

Simon Williams, writing of the vicissitudes of mind–body dualism across the illness trajectory, puts forward the argument that chronic illness sharpens our awareness of a 'normal' state of embodiment, and that consequently the ensuing struggle between states of 'dys-embodiment' (embodiment within a damaged or traumatised body) and efforts at re-embodiment fundamentally transform previous concepts of the body, the self and society (1996: 23; see also Hepworth, this volume). The extent to which individuals either identify with or react against the state of dys-embodiment to which chronic illness might lend itself reflects upon their acceptance or otherwise of the sick role which they feel they have been allocated. That this sick role is, to a considerable extent, a social construct in no way diminishes its force as a discourse upon the self. It constitutes, essentially, a binary vision of embodiment, one in which the sick and the healthy body dwell in often uncomfortable and paradoxical relation to each other. A similar vision of the essential difference between the world of the sick and the world of the well is addressed by Sontag in the introduction to her book *Illness as Metaphor* (1991: 3): 'Illness is the night-side of life, a more onerous citizenship. Everyone who is born holds dual citizenship, in the kingdom of the well and in the kingdom of the sick.'

In the case of John Diamond's account of his cancer (1998), a collection of articles in *The Times* newspaper, edited and collated into an extended narrative, this dys-embodiment and re-embodiment is presented as a continuing dialogue between the personae of Diamond as a columnist and cancer patient, and his readership. He uses the second person form to address the reader in his book just as he does in his column, which engenders a familiarity and involvement with the processes which Diamond describes in often absorbing detail.

In his account, Diamond rejects, indeed, 'despises' the military metaphors of illness, those ubiquitous references to battle or war against cancer famously criticised by Sontag. Why, he argues, should we accept this medically imposed model, which 'is based upon a morality which says that only those who fight hard against their cancer survive it or deserve to survive it – the corollary being that those who lose the fight deserved to do so?' (1998: 10). He conceives of his writing as an integral part of his 'cure', joining others who would see their intimate accounts of illness, diagnosis, treatment and relapse as therapeutic at least, and at best, revelatory.

Throughout the book, and in the film that covers the same period of his life, Diamond returns again and again to the question of his identity as a person with cancer, and how that identity is reconstituted through illness. He reminds us that his voice is the most recognisable item of his identity as a radio journalist, and with the particular cancer from which he suffers his voice becomes absent: in fact his tongue, as he muses sardonically, the metonym of language, is the very host to his cancer. He resents the new inarticulate identity that has been forced on him. He is compelled to write things down instead. He wakens from the first bout of surgery to be asked by the nurse: 'How do you feel?' In response, he scrawls on his clipboard the words: 'Absolutely fucking marvellous. And you?' His entire sense of identity, as he understands it, is deconstructed by the invasive and arduous treatments that he endures. He comments shortly after his departure from hospital after the first surgery, against medical advice, 'I didn't enjoy the person I now was', and 'I was not now the person my friends befriended, my wife married' (1998: 169–70).

The episodes which concern the ways in which Diamond sees himself as being *re-figured* by his cancer constitute, for the purposes of this chapter, the most remarkable aspect of the TV film. For example, in one scene, Diamond produces the notion of the 'other' as a transformative process that takes place within the self, describing how he has, in his own words, been delivered of a new, unwelcome identity, emphasising this otherness with the words: 'I really am not me.' More specifically, Diamond names the impostor who has 'taken him over' as 'a little old man called Albert or Norman or George'. This refiguration embodies his new identity as cancer patient, foregrounding the immediate consequences of treatment: the ruined voice, the indignity of feeding himself with a large soup-filled syringe, and the self-deprecatory dialogue that Diamond sustains for parts of the programme. In these passages, Diamond emphasises his sense of stigma, of being a 'dribbling, honking' outcast.

Diamond also talks at some length about his 'new voice': voice being an essential part of his identity as a broadcaster, of course, but also, within the frame of the cancer narrative, *voice is the explicit manifestation of the embodied nature of illness.* He talks of the inability of people who speak to him about his illness to accept this projection of the 'other' that he confronts them with, and the way in which they dismiss his illness as a way of refuting both otherness and the possibility of his (and ultimately, their own) death. Following this, the surgeon who has operated on Diamond emphasises the importance in 'this case' of obtaining maximum excision of the cancerous cells, not simply because this is the routine way of ensuring maximum protection against the cancer's return but because his voice is so central to Diamond's career and identity.

Perhaps the most startling image in the television film takes place when Diamond, after playing with his small children in the garden of his London home, tries on the radiation mask with which he has to be fitted at each visit for radiotherapy. Lying down on the grass, he positions the mask over his face, joking that it might enable its wearer to 'star in a German sado-masochism movie'. But it is not the joke as such which draws our attention, but rather the symbolically charged presence of the mask itself, acting as a provisional and necessary barrier between Diamond's 'true' face and the world. It is as if the illness had procured for him a new face, mapping precisely on to the old one and replacing it with this surrogate, just as his new, unwelcome identity causes him to reflect that 'I really am not me.' The idea of a stigmatised identity could not be more forcefully realised than through this remodelling of the face into an artefact, whose sinister appearance imbues its wearer not only with the grotesque appearance that serves Diamond's joke, but that, at the same time, protects his face (his 'true' identity) against the harmful radiation by directing it, through a number of lacerations and holes, towards the source of the cancer inside his mouth.

In his work on *Stigma* (1968), Goffman examined the distinction between the image that people have of themselves (their 'virtual social identity') and the way that other people see them (their 'actual social identity'). People with stigmas (attributes that have been labelled as deeply discrediting) confront problems in social interaction with 'normals' (Goffman's term) which can have particularly damaging consequences for their self-identity. If stigmatised individuals try to 'pass' as 'normal' they risk encountering a discrepancy between their own perceived virtual identity and their actual social identity. John Diamond, in his short demonstration of the radiation mask in the garden, confirms this distinction, taking it one step further. In the scenario described, it is not the perception of others that constitutes a conflict between his 'perceived' and his 'actual' social identity, but his own. He is, he tells us, no longer familiar with the person he has become, or is forced into becoming, both by the assaults of the treatment on his physical body and the concomitant re-figuration of himself that he construes from it. He is caught in limbo between a version of himself with which he is familiar, and one that he himself stigmatises (causing him to refer to himself in such self-deprecating terms as a 'dribbling, honking outcast'; 'doing an underwater impression of Charles Laughton'), and to liken his own appearance to a socially excluded figure, an actor in a sado-masochism film.

This stigmatised identity is mirrored in Marilyn French's account of her experience of living with cancer of the oesophagus, a cancer with an extremely low survival rate, when the author describes her loss of hair through chemotherapy, reporting that she 'felt like a leper, as if my limbs were shriveling and dropping off' (1998: 71). French also describes her mental state in terms reminiscent of Diamond's 'I really am not me.' She says: 'I was not inside myself', an almost perfect encapsulation of Williams's dys-embodiment. A person who is 'not inside herself' is (presumably) absent, elsewhere, consigned to an anonymous otherness. While this bears comparison with a Durkheimian *anomie* it remains more specific: the illness is personalised and owned. The 'person' is not to be found within the body, or, paraphrasing John Diamond's phrase, the person inside the body is no longer the one it once was.

Like Diamond, French reacts against the dominant metaphors of militancy – in particular the frequently encountered references to making war against cancer, attacking and destroying it (an attitude which does not extend to the publishers of her book, however, whose cover blurb refers to the author's 'successful battle against cancer'). She writes (1998: 85) 'I could not bear to think in terms of fighting ... because the thing I was supposed to fight was part of myself. So I visualized my white cells surrounding the cancer in an embrace and shrinking it, not in hate but as part of a natural process, transforming the cancer into something benign.' She writes about a friend with cancer who, she says, 'felt great bitterness toward her body for inflicting this terrible disease on her. She hated her body for it.' The woman who hates her own body for giving her cancer dies. French, meanwhile, although enduring an horrific ordeal through chemotherapy and undergoing a two-week coma as a consequence of her treatment, comes through, and this I suppose is the *telos* or goal of self-narrating, at least in the idealised sense – she returns to the present tense at the end of her story with a kind of grace. This return to the present, the reconciliation with narrative telos, is a prerequisite for any heroic journey. As we shall see, it is also a central proposition of Arthur Frank's work on illness narratives.

French makes another informative foray into the twinned identities of self and otherness in her book when she describes a visit to the oncology clinic by a pair of cosmetics saleswomen. She had signed up to attend this demonstration, for which the flyer promised the female cancer patients that they would be taught how to tie scarves 'to create an attractive head-covering', a relevant issue for those patients who had suffered hair loss through chemotherapy. They were, instead, given free bagfuls of cosmetics and had to endure a sales spiel from the two reps, who were 'young, shallow and criminally ignorant ... They had no training whatever in the effects of cancer on the human body' (1998: 74). French's tolerance is stretched to breaking point when 'a skinny, highly made-up young woman announced dramatically that "Eyebrows are *in* this year ladies"'. A ludicrous statement under any circumstances, French comments, but grotesquely insensitive when many of the women attending the demonstration had lost their eyebrows along with their hair (1998: 75). French sits disconsolately through the ninety-minute performance, and when she asks for a demonstration of head-coverings is told by the saleswomen that they know nothing about them. Here the true identity of the patients is seen to be salvageable or reparable, with the assistance of a consumer tradition that highlights and accentuates women's facial features (*cf.* Coupland, this volume), but is carried out in such a way as only to maximise the sense of difference already felt by the women patients. In attempting to impose a superficial modishness ('Eyebrows are *in* this year ladies') on a group whose absence of eyebrows is a mark of their otherness, the saleswomen only accentuate the dys-embodiment already implicit in the patients' condition.

Elsewhere, I have discussed the re-figuration of the patient through hair loss, emphasising its symbolic force (Gwyn, 1999; 2002) among children with cancer, and in this connection it is worth remembering that this re-figuration, while serving as a marker of cancer experience, has also been used (controversially) as an advertising strategy, in the 1997 advertisement for the Teenage Cancer Trust. The advertisement, which was circulated in newspapers and magazines during the winter of 1997–8, shows the reflection of a young woman with no hair, making her face up with lipstick in a mirror, underscored by the words *'Keeping up appearances is important. Even to a teenage girl with cancer.'* The advertisement misses the point (perhaps by straining to show its 'open-mindedness') that a discourse of 'appearances' cannot be limited to the token artefacts of cosmetics and that in presenting the image of the bald teenage girl as one stigmatised by her loss of hair, the advertisement surreptitiously colludes in that very process of stigmatisation. As Deborah Lupton (1997) argues, the dignity of the patient is ever under threat from the way that others, especially powerful others, are involved in constructing a new identity for them. She quotes forcefully from a woman talking about the symbolic value of hair loss: 'I couldn't explain to [the specialists] that there was a point beyond which I could not go. I didn't want to become hospitalised, I didn't want to become medicalised. I still wanted my dignity. They became fixated on the fact that I kept saying that I didn't want to lose my hair. But the hair was just a symbol of what I would be losing. It was – I didn't want to turn into a poor thing. I didn't want to be dependent. I didn't want to be bleating to friends, "Please help me"' (1997: 379).

There also exist, perhaps more emphatically, scenarios in which loss of a part of the body can be seen as emblematic in the face of the simplistic and dehumanising metaphors of consumerism. We might consider Frank's story (1995: 121) from Audre Lorde (1980) who is told by the nurse at her surgeon's office that not wearing a breast prosthesis is 'bad for the morale of the office'. The demands to adhere to a normative body shape was also the subject of an article in the British newspaper the *Guardian*, (*Guardian Review* 19 September 1998: 6–7). In this article a woman describes her decision not to camouflage the loss of her breast after surgery for cancer:

> At the time of my operation, I asked if I could have both breasts removed, but was told that the hospital didn't remove healthy breasts, which seemed extraordinary as they were happy to go to great expense recreating the bosom you once had. I could never have gone for reconstruction. The image of pink lumps of silicone in one's coffin filled me with panic.
>
> But it wasn't just queasiness that put me off. There is something creepy about the premise that you have to have two breasts to be complete and the idea that the experience of breast cancer can be 'covered up', as if it never happened, and women can be remade so they are almost as good as new. Who, I wonder, are we protecting? Ourselves or everyone else?

Such stories highlight the need of some individuals to protect and even display a spoiled identity, something which is analogous, according to Frank, to members of self-help recovery groups displaying their affiliation in the form of lapel badges. Audre Lorde pursues the mastectomy further, into a fantasy of identification with the Amazon warriors of Dahomey. She weaves aspects of her own identity as a black, one-breasted lesbian into this allegory of the initiation of Amazon warriors who had one breast cut off the better to shoot a bow. According to Frank, 'This metaphor joins her post-mastectomy body to her earlier black, lesbian, feminist self. The power of the metaphor is to give the mastectomy a kind of retrospective necessity: she had to lose a breast to become the full version of what she was before, but then only incompletely' (1995: 130). In other words, Lorde has become empowered by the full knowledge and the now embodied scars of her own metaphoric identity (cf. Woodward, Chapter 11 in this volume).

Arthur Frank relates this, and other stories of refiguration through cancer, to the narrative structure of the journey myth described by Joseph Campbell in his epic study of heroic journeys in world myths (1993). This journey myth maps well on to French's story, and even though Diamond presents himself very much as anti-hero (namely the 'coward' of his subtitle) his story, too, follows the quest plot, though ultimately a tragically curtailed one.[1] Campbell's description of the hero's journey is reducible to three stages: first *departure*, which begins with a call. This might be the symptom, the lump, dizziness, a cough. In John Diamond's story it is a phone call from his wife telling him that the oncologist has discovered cancer cells in his biopsy – all this while he is watching *Eastenders* on TV, a key moment in which the familiar world is transformed. In Marilyn French's account, departure is dealt with in rather a different way: she has to 'fight' for her diagnosis, to 'prod and nag' the doctors for more information, and eventually 'wrenches' the diagnosis from reluctant physicians (1998: 23). But the naming and locating of the cancer brings with it a certain relief, making treatment a positive event, which she likens to a reward.

After crossing the threshold into the world of the sick, the hero begins a second stage: *initiation*. According to Frank, tellers of quest stories use the metaphor of initiation implicitly and explicitly. Among the explicit ways by which this might be achieved I would include Marilyn French's account of the meetings of her 'coven', a group of her women friends who meet regularly during her illness, wear matching necklaces and go through various rituals and supplications for her, but the implicit initiation is surely the initiation into the vast marquee of technomedicine with all its obscure ritual and symbolism, one to which both French and Diamond claim they owed their lives, but which demands a full subservience to its own rites of initiation. Indeed, the anthropologist Robert Murphy refers to the illness experience and the medical worlds into which it leads as 'no less strange than the jungles he traveled in to do research' (Frank, 1995: 130).

Campbell refers to initiation as the road of trials – which in the illness story include all the sufferings, physical and emotional, that the patient endures. So for example, as we have seen, Diamond plays around with the grotesque plastic mask, likening it to a prop in a movie, but one which he must put over his own face for radiotherapy sessions in order to get better. This *initiation* period in a significant way underpins the subsequent unfolding of plot, the bedrock of narrative structure, since in the quest narrative the hero undergoes transformation, which is in fact crucial to the hero's attaining of responsibility. In addition, quest stories of illness, according to Frank, 'imply that the teller has been given something by the experience, usually some insight that must be passed on to others' (1995: 118). Of course, there are many cancer patients who do not respond to their illness experience in this way: they might simply retreat within the sick role, or conversely, attempt to ignore the illness and continue with their lives as best they can without care or treatment, both stances which, in their contrary ways, fulfil the criteria that Herzlich (1973) categorised collectively as 'Illness as destructive'. Whatever the route chosen, the market for accounts of illness experience is apparently insatiable, and the kinds of accounts we are currently examining represent only a tiny sample of the growing number of books being written by people with chronic illness, some of whom will be marketed as 'survivors' (like French), while others, like Ruth Picardie (1998) and John Diamond, will be remembered for having tracked the desperate terminal stages of their own diseases. That there has grown up a book-trade about terminal illness is by no means pleasing to all. Decca Aitkenhead, for example, a British journalist, broke a major taboo by referring to narratives of illness, death and dying as 'emotional pornography' (1998), but such views appear to be in the minority, or at least, if held, are not generally expressed in quite such abrasive terms.

Illness as a type of initiation represents citizenship of the 'kingdom of the sick', a place that many would rather not visit, let alone have foisted upon them. But the notion of illness as initiation is by no means a new idea, and relates to a commonly held conviction about the link between creativity and disease (Sandblom, 1982). Rooted in the Romantic tradition, this concept pervades Western art of the past two centuries. It is this perspective that Herzlich (1973) terms 'Illness as Liberator', and that subscribes to a belief in growth through suffering, granting insights into one's own life and greater lucidity and awareness of questions relating to life and death. Such an attitude is most obviously apparent in the hypochondriac labours of a writer such as Proust.

The issue of initiation held particular significance for DiGiacamo (1987), who, because of her profession as anthropologist and her enforced role as patient, placed her ambiguously as 'an anthropologist in the kingdom of the sick'. Having being diagnosed with

Hodgkin's disease, DiGiacomo at first approached her doctors as colleagues rather than superiors. She was taken aback at their response to her: 'Generally their first reaction was surprise at my failure to defer to them, then disapproval. Occasionally, when I persisted, conflict resulted. These disagreements first prompted me to think of my relationships with my doctors in anthropological terms' (1987: 320). It is this attempt at questioning and realigning the roles within the clinic that provided DiGiacomo with her quest narrative; and the decision to remain 'an anthropologist in the kingdom of the sick' served as the guiding text for her 'initiation'. After an argument with the hospital's leading expert on Hodgkin's disease and a further confrontation with an 'unsmiling' anaesthetist, she finds herself labelled as a 'bad patient'. This, she argues, is because she appeared to question the established hospital routines, rationalised as being necessary for the efficient running of the hospital and the good of the patient. She was kept uninformed about the course and, to a large extent, the nature of her treatment, and when summoned to the hospital without advance notice for the first dose of treatment, she again contravened the expected sick role by refusing to attend until a more convenient time. Once in treatment, she antagonises the radiologist by referring to her radiation burns as burns, rather than using the correct formula of 'a radiation *reaction*'. When she retorts that it is quite obviously a burn, since her skin is burnt and blistered, the radiologist answers: 'we don't call it that'. Further confrontation regarding her hair loss and an evident falsehood relayed to her by the radiologist cause her to reflect that doctors believe patients to be incapable of handling the truth, and that they must therefore be shielded from it (1987: 323). To a large extent, then, DiGiacomo's quest became her self-selected role as 'patient-researcher' (which to her medical carers, became more and more equated with simple non-compliance and membership of the 'awkward squad'). She describes yet further confrontations with oncologist and radiologist, and is yet again given a patronising lecture by the radiologist: 'We simply cannot explain everything to patients. We've found that they just can't absorb much information at any given time. And anyway this isn't a post-graduate course in radiology.'

Communication between departments at the hospital is shown to be dislocated and unreliable. Papers get lost, blood samples and X-rays are delivered to the wrong places. Information about dates and duration of treatment is never clear, and arrangements for her eventual discharge remain obscure. When she is eventually allowed to eat solids after seven days on a drip, she is fed fried eggs and orange juice, which cause further distress and vomiting. However, DiGiacomo's frequently hostile reaction to her hospitalisation and to the patronising attitude of medical personnel is not reproduced simply to vent her anger: she is attempting throughout to question and subvert the passive role of patient that she has been allocated, resisting the prescribed rites of initiation in favour of her own ethnographer's account of the operations of power and authority in a medical setting. Her 'initiation' becomes a programme of resistance to an imposed sense of patienthood. She concludes that to 'get angry, to assert oneself in the only way possible ... was to step out of one's assigned role, and thus to threaten the entire institution. Of all the transgressions a patient may commit, non-compliance is the worst' (1987: 326).

The third phase of Campbell's journey is the *return*. The storyteller returns as one who is no longer ill (but may be in remission), and yet who is marked by illness. The marked person lives in this world but is also denizen of another world: in Campbell's words, 'master of two worlds'. Again we are reminded of Sontag's dictum that we all hold citizenship of two parallel worlds. There is no simplistic or unifying bond between all survivors of life-threatening illness, of course; and among some commentators (John Diamond among them) little to be found within the experience of being ill that is any way 'beneficial'. But patients must necessarily wait for their full 'return' to normal life (or its near equivalent when carrying the trauma of long-term illness) and, of course, those, like Diamond and Picardie, who die, are denied this rounding-off of the journey. Marilyn French, towards the end of her account, questions the standard assumption that life is always better than death, since for many, this is simply not the case. And yet, she argues, there is an inherent 'clinging to life' even in the most forlorn circumstances, which, she claims, emanates from 'something deeper and grittier and more elemental' (1998: 249). Later, she reflects on the transformative power of chronic illness in a way that resonates with Campbell's concept of 'Return':

[A] serious illness or disaster is transforming. It changes not just our bodies and psyches but the context of desire. The field from which we choose our desires shifts under our feet; we choose differently, not just because we have changed but because we see different elements to choose among. For me, the change has been profound: I am happier than I have ever been, despite my handicaps.

(French, 1998: 253)

Furthermore, the citizenship of both worlds which French carries with her allows her the authority to speak of the experience of having lived through and survived the one, and apply the knowledge that she gained therefrom to the other: 'I am happy that sickness, if it had to happen, brought me to where I am now. It is a better place than I have been before. I am grateful to have been allowed to live long enough to experience it' (1998: 255).

Whatever the routes through illness and suffering, the principal role of the storyteller in these narratives is that of witness. As such it corresponds well with Frank's notion of the 'communicative body' (1995: 127), an idealised and idealising status whereby the sick person returns to the world of the healthy with a gift: 'the communicative body seeks to share the boon that it has gained upon its own return. Others need this boon for the journeys they necessarily will undertake.' Thus the illness experience becomes mythologised and allows the survivor-witness to achieve a kind of grace, which, on return, is no longer uniquely theirs but may be shared with others.

The final question I want to address is how we do social science in the ambiguous zone between autobiographical writing and reflexive ethnography such as we find when social scientists such as Frank, DiGiacomo, Zola (1982) and Murphy (1987) produce their autobiographical accounts. Obviously not all social scientists are going to have life-threatening illnesses, and of those that do, not all are going to want to write up their experiences as social science. But DiGiacomo (1987; 1992), I believe, helped show the way in which this can be done. Throughout her illness and its treatment she regarded her profession of anthropologist as a lens through which to study the process of cancer care and her own subjective response to it. However difficult this proved and however problematic this dual persona proved for some of the doctors who treated her, she adhered to a strategy whereby the meaning and consequences of her own experience were not divorced from her professional role as ethnographer. She became, in her own terms, a 'credible witness' (1992: 132), receiving and refuting *en route* comments from her doctors such as: 'I don't think it's wise for you to try to become an expert on your own disease, it could be very damaging psychologically' (1987: 321). DiGiacomo saw her own work as, in part, a rewriting of the social text 'given' to cancer patients, and, in the tradition of constructionism, social science must be that or else be nothing but the provision of answers to unasked questions. Or in her own words: '"Ethnographic practice" must come to mean not only how we do our fieldwork and construct ethnographic texts, but how we live our lives' (1992: 132). Researchers into language and culture might question the conflation of the individual's subjective experience with his or her professional research, but as DiGiacomo points out, those of us who work within the fields of medical anthropology (or, I would add, any other area of social science) need to recognise that the mind–body dichotomy so central to a Western understanding of health issues 'is but a variant of a more deeply rooted and pervasive dichotomy, that of subject and object' ... which also gives rise to the Self-Other distinction in ethnographic research' (1992: 133).

Ellis and Bochner (1999) call for bringing a greater expression of emotion and personal narrative into medical social science. They argue as follows: 'To move in the direction of a narrative, evocative, medical sociology, is to give more room to the sense-making struggles of people whose illusions of prediction and control have been interrupted by illness or death. The move requires that we re-evaluate the idea of neutrality and admit that what we write happens not only to other people but also to ourselves' (1999: 235). This commitment to an involved, involving and compassionate social science is obviously bound to elicit opposition, and that, too, is worthwhile, so long as the resistance to narrativisation and the expression of emotion in academic writing is not expressed in purely oppositional terms; in other words, that its opponents do not believe their science to be sanctioned by an intrinsically more accurate, objectivist grasp of social reality.

Perhaps the most interesting lesson to be learned from much of the current autobiographical writing on illness experience is that the dichotomy of mind–body also has its corollary in the dichotomy of thought–emotion in academic discourse. Just as scholarly writing is mentalistic, rational and controlled, so the productions of revelatory autobiographical writing, because of their profound subjectivity, are frequently considered to be outside the realm of serious social science. As Rosaldo commented in her blueprint study for an anthropology of self and feeling, 'bursts of feeling will continue to be opposed to careful thought' (1984: 137). As long as academic writing maintains this dualistic attitude of clear thought versus muddled emotion we shall be forced to consider an 'emotional' life as being utterly separated from (or inimical to) an 'intellectual' life.

Illness narrative might be seen as an ideal way of studying the expression of embodied thought, a way of forging the kind of borderline writing, poised between literature and ethnography, espoused by anthropologists such as Clifford and Marcus (Clifford and Marcus, 1986; Clifford, 1997; Marcus, 1998). One way into this challenging discipline could well be, as Williams suggests, to focus upon narratives of embodiment relating to disease and disorder, which provide a 'conceptual bridge between a phenomenological approach to embodiment, and a broader consideration of the socially constructed nature of illness and the cultural scripts of sickness' (1996: 42). Until this is done, we shall be consigned to a version of health communication that, under the control of a powerful and remote professional elite, still (after a quarter-century of 'patient-centred medicine') dichotomises mind and body, intellect and emotion, subject and object, selfhood and otherness, health and sickness, rather than seeing one as always implicit within the other.

Note

1. Although John Diamond was in remission from his illness when this paper was delivered at the Round Table Conference in July 1999, he died on 2 March 2001 before the final draft of the chapter was completed.

References

Aitkenhead, D. (1998) 'Before They Say Goodbye'. *The Modern Review*. 4 February: 32–7.

Campbell, J. (1993) [1949] *The Hero with a Thousand Faces*. London: Fontana.

Clifford, J. (1997) *Routes: Travel and Translation in the Late Twentieth Century*. Cambridge, MA: Harvard University Press.

Clifford, J. and Marcus, G. (1986) *Writing Culture: the Poetics and Politics of Ethnography*. Berkeley, CA: University of California Press.

Diamond, J. (1998) *C: Because Cowards Get Cancer Too … .* London: Vermillion.

DiGiacomo, S. (1987) 'Biomedicine as a Cultural System: An Anthropologist in the Kingdom of the Sick'. In H.A. Baer (ed.) *Encounters with Biomedicine: Case Studies in Medical Anthropology*. New York: Gordon & Breach.

DiGiacomo, S. (1992) 'Metaphor as Illness: Postmodern Dilemmas in the Representation of Body, Mind and Disorder'. *Medical Anthropology* 14: 109–37.

Ellis, C. and Bochner, A. (1999) 'Bringing Emotion and Personal Narrative into Medical Social Science'. *Health* 3(2): 229–37.

Frank, A. (1995) *The Wounded Storyteller*. Chicago: University of Chicago Press.

French, M. (1998) *A Season in Hell*. London: Virago.

Geertz, C. (1988) *Works and Lives: the Anthropologist As Author*. Stanford, CA: Stanford University Press.

Gergen, K. (1994) *Realities and Relationships*. Cambridge MA: Harvard University Press.

Goffman, E. (1968) *Stigma: Notes on the Management of Spoiled Identity*. Harmondsworth: Penguin.

Gwyn, R. (1999) 'Captain of My Own Ship: Metaphor and the Discourse of Chronic Illness'. In L. Cameron and G. Low (eds) *Researching and Applying Metaphor*. Cambridge: Cambridge University Press.

Gwyn, R. (2002) *Communicating Health and Illness*. London: Sage.

Hass, R. (1989) *Human Wishes*. New York: The Ecco Press.

Herzlich, C. (1973) *Health and Illness*. London: Academic Press.

Josselson, R. and Lielich, A. (1996) *Making Meaning of Narratives*. Thousand Oaks: Sage.

Lorde, A. (1980) *The Cancer Journals*. San Francisco, CA: Aunt Lute Books.

Lupton, D. (1997) 'Consumerism, Reflexivity and the Medical Encounter'. *Social Science and Medicine* 45(3): 373–81.

Marcus, G. (1998) *Ethnography Through Thick and Thin*. Princeton, NJ : Princeton University Press, 1998.

Murphy, R. (1987) *The Body Silent*. New York: Henry Holt.

Paget, M.A. (1995) 'Performing the Text'. In J. Van Maanen (ed.) *Representation in Ethnography*. Thousand Oaks: Sage.

Picardie, R. (1998) *Before I Say Goodbye*. Harmondsworth: Penguin.

Rosaldo, M. (1984) 'Toward an Anthropology of Self and Feeling'. In R.A. Shweder and R.A. LeVine (eds) *Culture Theory: Essays on Mind, Self and Emotion*. Cambridge: Cambridge University Press, 137–57.

Sandblom, P. (1982) *Creativity and Disease: How Illness Affects Literature, Art and Music*. New York: Marion Boyars.

Sontag, S. (1991) *Illness as Metaphor/AIDS and its Metaphors*. Harmondsworth: Penguin.

Williams, S. (1996) 'The Vicissitudes of Embodiment Across the Chronic Illness Trajectory'. *Body & Society*. 2(2): 23–47.

Zola, I. (1982) *Missing Pieces: a Chronicle of Living with a Disability*. Philadelphia: Temple University Press.

11
The Statistical Body

Kathleen Woodward

> Once you have had cancer, the chance of having it again is
> even greater than before.
>
> Jane Lazarre, *Wet Earth and Dreams* (121)

> Probability and statistics crowd in upon us ... There are more
> explicit statements of probabilities presented on American
> prime time television than explicit acts of violence ... Our
> public fears are endlessly debated in terms of probabilities:
> chances of meltdowns, cancers, muggings, earthquakes,
> nuclear winters, AIDS, global greenhouses, what next? There is
> nothing to fear (it may seem) but the probabilities themselves.
>
> Ian Hacking, *The Taming of Chance* (4–5)

I

If we live in a visual culture where society is distinguished by the spectacle, we also live in the society of the statistic.[1] Images of the body are
circulated endlessly in postmodern culture. Figures of the body are also
continuously deployed in the discourse of statistics as a way of understanding our lives and comparing ourselves to others. Statistics are the
very atmosphere we breathe, the strange weather in which we live, the
continuous emission of postmodern media life. Body statistics are
transmitted at every moment of the day and night – on the Internet, in
the newspaper and magazines, and on TV and the radio. Statistics tell
us how many African-Americans hold management positions in the
financial district in New York; how many Asians make up the student
body at the University of California; how many people over 65 are
employed full-time. Statistics such as these are based on what I call
'difference demographics'. Statistics also stream from the worlds of
sports and beauty. We learn about baseball batting averages and yards

rushed in football; about how many men and women are having cosmetic surgery; about the reduction in the appearance of face wrinkles if a certain cream is used (see Coupland, this volume).

Of all the statistics that call up figures of the body, an extremely large proportion have to do with the vulnerable body – with disease and ill-being, accidents and violence, and ultimately death. Examples are to be found everywhere. 'Every year, congestive heart failure contributes to about 300,000 deaths in the United States', we learn in an article entitled 'Next Frontiers' in the 25 June 2001 issue of *Newsweek*, 'which is nearly twice as many as stroke and seven times as many as breast cancer' (44). Ninety people on death row in America's prisons have been declared innocent since 1973, a statistic that has led many to call for an end to the death penalty. 'One out of three women over 40 experience it', declares an advertisement for Serenity Thin Pads in the August 2001 issue of *Good Housekeeping*; 'The issue of bladder control' (17). On 1 August 2001, CNN Headline News reported that eighteen high school and college football players have died of heatstroke deaths in the United States since 1995. These statistics profiling the body are unsettling. Melancholy. Grim.

Statistics hail us in the Althusserian sense. Along with the anecdote, the statistic is one of the pervasive narrative conventions of postmodern media culture. Statistics frequently open what is called a 'story' in print, broadcast or internet news, to be followed by an anecdote – or vice versa. Indeed, statistics in and of themselves often constitute the story and our imaginations supply a corresponding anecdote or scenario. In the United States, for instance, we learned in 1997 from our then Secretary of Health and Human Services that domestic violence accounts for 20 to 30 per cent of the visits to emergency rooms by women.[2] Here statistics are themselves the deep structure and manifest content of the story, numerological protagonists that stalk their potential victims. Here a narrative has been compacted into the most minimal and impersonal of fragments – a statistic. Injury by abuse is the story, and female readers may find themselves imagining what might happen if their own partners turn angry with them.

Even when the citation of statistics is meant to provide reassurance, it may more often than not produce its opposite: a sense of foreboding and insecurity. Two other stories from 1997 are cases in point. In late 1997 it was widely reported that an older woman had died in air turbulence on a flight from Japan to Honolulu. The airline industry quickly released the following statistic, which was announced in turn by the media, in an effort to restore confidence so that we would soon forget any newly engendered fear of flying: only two people, we were told, had died of air turbulence over the last fifteen years. My informal and highly unscientific survey of friends and colleagues revealed that, instead of being comforted, many found themselves wondering about the circumstances of the death of that unidentified other person. How did he/she die? What happened? Where? When? They created the outlines of a narrative based on this single statistic and further, vaguely fantasised about their own possible future death from air turbulence, resolving always to keep their seat belts fastened to diminish any possible injury. On 30 December 1997, the headline bannered as its top news on CompuServe, an internet service provider, proclaimed: 'Homicide Rate Down in 1997'. This is a statistical variant on what Freud termed the declaration of desire by negation, although here it is not desire but the sense of being at risk that is announced. That the number of murders had declined was supposed to be good news. But there is no doubt that those fewer murders remained violent death sentences. Moreover, that the very subject of the sentence fragment is the homicide rate itself suggests that statistics, although an impersonal and implacable force, possess a peculiar fateful agency akin to that of the ancient Greek gods. Being reduced to a statistic, as we say, is definitely not a fate to be desired.

In cases such as these a pervasive habit of mind is to take a statistic about the past or present and extrapolate it into the future, in the process often creating a scenario of harm to the body or, at the extreme, mortality. I find this fascinating and thus my focus in this chapter will be on the statistics of the vulnerable body as a discourse of *probability* rather than as one used to make sense of the past or of the present. Statistics: it is the science that, according to the definition given in the 1987 *Random House College Dictionary of the English Language,* 'deals with the collection, classification, analysis, and interpretation of numerical facts or data, and that, by use of mathematical theories of probability, imposes order and regularity on aggregates of more or less disparate elements'. By means of statistical probability, then, predictability is assigned to a large number of 'more or less disparate elements', to a vast array of what are, in fact, different bodies. In this sense, statistics are probabilities cast, much as are dice, into possible and alternative futures, and these futures of the vulnerable body often take on a dark dimension.[3] Statistical probabilities of the vulnerable body seem to implicate us as individuals in scenarios of disaster by disease, accident and violence in an abstraction expressed by the ultimate abstraction – numbers. The key word here is risk.

From this perspective it is statistics, rather than economics, that should be known as the dismal science. For statistics is a science that is now circulated interminably in everyday life as a discourse of risk. We are at risk, it seems, of anything and everything. 'The more women a man has sex with, the higher his risk of developing prostate cancer in middle age', reported the *New York Times* on 17 July 2001. 'By far the most powerful risk factor for osteoarthritis', John L. Zenk announced in *Total Health* in 2001, 'is age. It is estimated that 68 per cent of individuals older than age 55 and over 80 per cent of people older than 75 have osteoarthritis' (64). Our bodies are figured as being in a perpetual state of risk. Of death by mad cow disease. Of high cholesterol. Of toxic waste. Of crossing the street. Of rape. Of hormone replacement therapy. Of crushing a finger with a hammer.[4]

In the immediate aftermath of the 11 September 2001 destruction of the twin towers of the World Trade Center in New York, the discourse of risk at the hands of terrorist attacks was omnipresent in the United States, with the emphasis falling on bioterrorism (anthrax, small pox, typhus), threats targeted specifically at the body, not at property or symbolic structures. How to allay the public's panic? It should come as no surprise that one of the chief ways was to counter the (hopefully) statistically minimal threat of bodily harm from terrorism with the deployment of statistics of risk from everyday life in post-industrial society. Consider this excerpt from a piece by Jane Brody that appeared in the *New York Times* on 9 October 2001: 'the current focus on potential acts of terrorism is diverting people from responding to real and immediate risks to their well-being, and in some cases prompting them to take real risks because they are so busy avoiding hypothetical ones'. The real risks are those encountered every day – 'a plateful of steak,' 'cigarette smoking' – with the risks from terrorism reduced to the 'hypothetical'. What does Brody single out as her first example? 'A case in point: driving long distances instead of flying. On a per-mile basis, flying is much safer, even in these uncertain times. Each year, tens of thousands of people are killed on the roads, whereas the annual number of airplane deaths almost never exceeds a few hundred, as was the case even on Sept. 11' (D6).

As the sociologist Ulrich Beck has persuasively argued, industrial society has been succeeded by the risk society. To figure the modern, Walter Benjamin imagined a visionary 'angel of history' who, although turned toward the future, in fact faces the past and the 'wreckage' wrought by catastrophe (1969: 25). Today we face a future figured as statistical risk, with wreckage everywhere dispersed into the years that lie ahead. Ultimately, as the philosopher Ian Hacking has suggested, in the end what we may have come to fear is not a specific thing – any *thing* – but rather probability itself, the future. What we fear is risk itself.

Rather than anchoring us to a stable life-world, then, statistics that forecast the future of our bodies engender insecurity in the form of low-grade intensities that, like low-grade fevers, permit us to go about our everyday lives but in a state of statistical stress. In the risk society we adopt, for example, the stance of medical self-surveillance, monitoring our own vital statistics even as we listen to the nation's own medical statistics routinely announced by governmental agencies. Statistical stress (and statistical boredom, which is related to it) can thus be understood as a particular structure of feeling in Raymond Williams's (1977) sense, one that discloses the society of the statistic in which we live today, a mediatised, marketised, and medicalised culture in which the notion of being at risk has assumed dominant proportions. There is something both strangely unnerving and numbing in this phenomenon of statistical stress, a structure of feeling that produces risk as a commodity and then offers goods and services to assuage that same sense of stress.

The effect accompanying catastrophic statistical discourse about large-scale concerns – population growth, for example, or terrorism – is highly unstable; what at one moment may impress us as urgent may in the next seem simply boring. But when our own individual futures are at stake, statistical stress can turn into panic and strike with compelling and sustained force, increasing exponentially in intensity. Statistical panic: fatally, we feel that a certain statistic, which is in fact based on an aggregate and is only a measure of probability, actually represents our very future.[5] Such panic is usually fleeting. Based as it is on a number, it usually cannot be endured for long. Moreover, in virtually all cases, it will surely be drowned out by another number (one's risk will be recalculated on the basis of a new study). Yet a given statistic can also come to drastically colour our very lives.

How do we survive into the future in the postmodern society of risk? For some, it would seem, by eliminating as much risk as possible. By understanding every day as one in which our ability is tested to survive not only actual threats (a hold-up at gunpoint in the city, for instance), but also the invisible atmosphere that everywhere radiates risk, projecting it far into the future. As the philosopher Zygmunt Bauman has so aptly suggested, the 'postmodern strategy of survival' is to slice 'time (all of it, exhaustively, without residue) into short-lived, evanescent

episodes. It rehearses mortality, so to speak, by practicing it day by day'
(1992: 29). Our daily work – our career, in the sociologist Erving
Goffman's sense – is to manage our futures in terms of avoiding risk.
But there are other strategies as well, as I hope the following discussion
of three recent illness narratives in which the statistical medical body
figures prominently will make clear: a breast cancer narrative from the
primetime television medical drama *Chicago Hope* that was broadcast in
December 1997 on CBS in the United States, Yvonne Rainer's 1996
feature-length film *MURDER and murder*, which explores the disturbing
discrepancy between the scientific language of statistics and their experiential dimension in relation to breast cancer, and the historian Alice
Wexler's *Mapping Fate*, a memoir published in 1995 that engages the
experience of being at risk for Huntington's disease.

II

In one of the narrative lines in the 1997 episode from *Chicago Hope*, a
middle-aged woman – she is a wife and mother of two children –
insists to a young male surgeon that she wants a double mastectomy.
The surgeon is not only reluctant to do the operation, he is horrified,
because she does not in fact have breast cancer. But, as she explains,
she has an 86 per cent chance of getting breast cancer (this statistic is
based solely on family history; her mother died of breast cancer and
her two sisters also died of breast cancer). For her the statistic is like an
oncoming train that she must avoid at all costs. Although the statistic
is an abstraction and is not linked to a certain outcome, it has for her a
galvanising force. Here we so clearly see the difference between the
scientific use of the language of risk and its experiential dimension:
this fictional woman's experience of the feeling of being at risk – or
what I am calling statistical panic – discloses a terrifying future: for her
it is the absolute certainty that her life will be cut short by disease.[6]
Thus the immaterial social technology of the statistical discourse of risk
has a tangible effect on her body and her psyche.

The doctor's initial reaction is that the woman is suffering from para-
noia and hysteria, two emotions that are assuredly not associated with
rational decision-making. But in the end he is persuaded by her unwa-
vering determination and the gravity of her statistical prognosis to
perform the operation (along the way he also gets a lesson from the
woman with whom he is romantically involved, learning that a
woman's sexual attractiveness should not be irrevocably linked with
her breasts and that love should triumph over such dramatic bodily

change). What to the surgeon at first seems an insane course of action is disclosed in the course of the narrative as pre-eminently rational in an unequivocally calculating sense. If we generally regard statistics as a depersonalising force, here we see that when we apply them to ourselves, creating our own emotional dramas out of them, they can have an overwhelming power, orienting us to the world in a particular way, focusing our attention on eliminating risk by confronting it as a certainty, as an absolute and not as a probability. In order to avoid being reduced to a statistic, which in this case would entail a death sentence, this fictional character from *Chicago Hope* uses her panic as energy to guide the surgeon's knife to her breasts and thus to obliterate altogether – or so she thinks – her risk of such cancer.

The narrative is designed to persuade us, along with the surgeon, that her decision is 'rational'. Her clearly defined role as a wife and mother is represented as the maintenance of her health at all costs. The all-powerful protagonist of the story is the figure of risk: she has an 86 per cent chance of developing breast cancer. Interestingly enough, however, the fact that her panic carries with it a financial price as well as an emotional price is never mentioned. The surgeon is carefully represented as never lobbying in any way for the operation, for which he would receive a fee (no doubt a big one). Instead he is firmly opposed to it and must be convinced to do it. The mutual entailment of the society of risk, which requires the production of statistics, and of consumer culture, is never suggested. The high figure of 86 per cent represents, as it were, the high cost of maximising this woman's health. In the healthcare system in the United States this carries a steep price tag and results, in cases such as these, in what I call the pricing of panic. For sustaining health has become a major preoccupation in contemporary consumer culture, one that relies upon statistical reports to increase demand for its products.[7] As Robin Bunton, Sarah Nettleton and Roger Burrows argue, 'At a cultural level "healthism" has become a central plank of contemporary consumer culture as images of youthfulness, vitality, energy and so on have become key articulating principles of a range of contemporary popular discourses' (1995: 1).

This episode from *Chicago Hope* is a clear instance of the medical melodrama, where public and private space intersect in the operating room, where fraught decisions are reduced to obvious choices, and where good motherhood is represented as taking a knife to the body and spending a lot of money in the process. In short, the address to women and the work of consumption are yet again aligned in the representational space of television. In this clear-cut melodramatic world, the wife (she is also, we remember, a mother of two) is presented from the beginning as unambivalent, as having no questions or qualms about her decision. But I would argue that the very experiential quality of statistical panic is that it carries uncertainty with it, an uncertainty intrinsic to it. The TV narrative is cast in black-and-white terms, as a debate between two competing and supremely confident positions. What in fact panics us, however, is that we cannot be certain of the future of our own unique bodies, however much, as in this case, epidemiologists have quantified the probabilities based on an aggregate of bodies for us. What is peculiarly reductive about this TV narrative is that the woman is never represented as hesitating over what she thinks she should do.

In her important essay 'The Meaning of Lumps: A Case Study of the Ambiguities of Risk', Sandra Gifford distinguishes between 'two distinct dimensions' of risk in a medical context: 'a technical, objective or *scientific* dimension and a socially experienced or *lived* dimension'. As she explains:

> although epidemiologists speak of risk as being a measured property of a group of people, clinicians speak of risk as a special property of an individual. Risk becomes something that the patient suffers; a sign of a future disease that the clinician can diagnose, treat and manage. For the patient, risk becomes a lived or experienced state of ill-health and a symptom of future illness ... These different dimensions of risk as understood and experienced by epidemiologists further blur the already ambiguous relationship between health and ill-health. This ambiguity results in the creation of a new state of being healthy and ill; a state that is somewhere between health and disease and that results in the medicalisation of a woman's life.
>
> (1986: 215)

The healthy woman from *Chicago Hope* is not represented as suffering risk but rather as managing it from a technical, objective or scientific point of view, a view that is skewed because her body is not a representative body, but merely one of a huge aggregate on which her statistical probability of contracting cancer is based. Moreover, the physician is at first sure that she should not have the operation; he does not interpret the risk the statistic implies for her but rather dismisses it. Thus, in this episode of *Chicago Hope*, the kind of ambiguity that Gifford so discerningly identifies is not represented. This is what accounts for my uneasiness with the narrative, my sense that the story is truly bizarre. How could we possibly allow a number to have such decisive and unambiguous power over us?

But the cultural injunction to avoid medical risk is all-pervasive. Phyllis Rose, a writer in her middle years, comments on this from the perspective of her own experience with possible breast cancer in *A Year of Reading Proust: A Memoir in Real Time*, published in 1997. Told by her doctor to have a breast biopsy done to test some small spots of calcification, she puts it off, judging that the odds of one in five were not overwhelming. Her friends are aghast and censorious. They think her frivolous and self-destructive. 'To cling to any personal preference, to value personal convenience in the face of a threat of cancer', Rose concludes, 'is to defy a culture style so widely approved that it has the force of wisdom and responsible practice ... Committed to having the biopsy, nevertheless I talked about it with a studied levity which to me signaled equanimity and mastery of my fate, but which to many of my friends bespoke shallowness, until, one day, talking to a good friend, I was reduced to tears and bewildered questions' (131). Here Rose was judged as being deficient because she was not suffering or displaying statistical panic. Her friends made what they thought was a moral judgement. As Solomon Katz and others have argued, we live in a culture where for many people moral concerns are associated not with religious tenets and values, but rather with illness and health; morality – what is referred to as 'secular morality' – in an instance such as this is based on calculations of risk emerging from the field of epidemiology.

Although this event receives only passing attention in *A Year of Reading Proust*, it is significant because Rose, unlike the fictional TV character from *Chicago Hope*, reflects critically on postmodern culture's circulation of the statistical body of risk. For another way that we survive into the future in our postmodern culture of risk is by dissecting the very deployment of statistical discourse and its effects upon us, by reflecting on our affective response to the language of risk. Importantly, in both Yvonne Rainer's *MURDER and murder* and Alice Wexler's *Mapping Fate*, probable statistical death is the underwriter of alternative futures. If *MURDER and murder* entertains the question of what statistical panic feels like, how it can get you in its steel grips, Wexler shows us how she finally resolved not to concede control to it.

Rainer's bold film *MURDER and murder* takes up the subjects of breast cancer, ageing, and love between two older women. For Rainer murder in capital letters (MURDER), as opposed to murder in lower case (murder), is death from clearly defined social causes and is thus death that could have been prevented – such as death caused by nuclear testing and DDT, death from homophobia and other forms of stigma. In what Rainer has herself termed the most psychologically realistic of her films, *MURDER and murder* contains a running commentary on statistics – thematically, literally, figuratively, and perhaps most courageously, autobiographically. *MURDER and murder* also thematises the possibility of seeing into the future. Ghosts of the characters when they were younger haunt the action that takes place in the present, commenting wistfully, wryly and even statistically on possible futures. As the young ghost of one of the two main characters says dreamily, 'Just think of it: if in one year only one girl from every graduating class in every high school in the country becomes a lesbian, that means 33,000 lesbians! In a decade that would add up to 330,000. And in thirty years it would be a million!' (101). Within the context of the film such an increase in lesbian bodies is a utopian prospect.

But what is foregrounded is a statistical nightmare of the female body. In the course of the narrative, the 63-year-old Mildred is diagnosed with breast cancer and undergoes a mastectomy. While the credits roll at the end of the film, she says in voice-over, referring to statistics specifically about lesbians and breast cancer, 'these statistics make me tired' (117). To which Doris, her younger partner replies, 'So many ways to get messed up. Your numbers are even more terrifying than mine.' Mildred: 'They're just numbers. Everyone has a different set of numbers. You can't live your life by numbers.' But, as I have been suggesting, we are virtually required by the society of the statistic to do so. And often for what we would term good reasons – acting in a manner in accordance with avoiding mortal disease, maximising our health. This is the position Doris takes. Doris to Mildred: 'But you can use the numbers as cautionary. Like, when did you last get a pap smear and mammogram?' If the tone is for a moment ironically light (fun is occasionally poked at statistics in the film), the implications of Mildred's answer are horrifying. 'Oh don' start on me now. I don' know, two or three years ago.' Two or three years ago! My first reaction is to wish that she had had a mammogram! I react like Phyllis Rose's friends, who castigate her for delaying the biopsy her physician had advised. (This is further complicated by the fact that having a mammogram provides no guarantee.) Then I remember: Mildred is a fictional character. But the final frame of the film returns the spectator to the sobering light of the real world before the film fades out. It reads:

IN MEMORIAM
NANCY GRAVES
SHIRLEY TRIEST.

Within the context of the film the deaths of these two real women seem to be statistical fatalities. Death by statistic. And by a horrible irony, the deaths of these women will in fact be reduced to statistics, data going into the aggregate to generate a new mix and new probabilities for the future of other women. Yet at the same time Rainer's film is dedicated to the memory of these women, to the meaning their lives held for other people, and is thus also a refusal to allow them to be reduced to statistics.

It has been said of some fictional narratives (of Thomas Hardy's late nineteenth-century novels, for example) that the landscape assumes the status of a character. In *MURDER and murder* statistics are both the environment in which these women live and an uncompromising force that is mercurial in nature. Even if you follow all the rules (you eat the 'right' food, you exercise, you don't live next to a toxic waste dump), you may be hit. Sobering if not frightening statistics appear as crawling titles across the bottom of the screen, accompanying much of the film. Here are some examples. *'There are 1.8 million women in the U.S. who've been diagnosed with breast cancer. One million others have the disease and do not yet know it'* (88). *'One out of four women who are diagnosed with breast cancer die within the first five years. Forty percent will be dead within ten years'* (89). In one scene, fragments of a statistic are stencilled on the wall and in another we see a statistic being carefully inscribed on another wall, as if it were graffiti. It reads, *'In 1992 thirty-seven and a half million people in the U.S. had no health insurance'* (112). In one of the most important sequences in *MURDER and murder*, statistics about breast cancer are stencilled on the canvas of a boxing ring, literally covering the floor on which Mildred and Doris first fight and then make love. Although statistics are omnipresent in contemporary culture, the profound effects they have upon us have largely been ignored. Thus one of the major achievements of *MURDER and murder* is to show how they constitute the very stage upon which we act out our lives. In *MURDER and murder* statistics are literally made visible.

Yvonne Rainer, a lesbian and in her early sixties when she made this film, appears as herself in *MURDER and murder*, interrupting the fictional narrative with her own autobiographical commentary. In the boxing ring scene I referred to above, she sits in the audience right in front of the ring. She is wearing a fighter's robe and at one point addresses the camera, slightly offside. She speaks in an even, almost toneless voice that verges on the deadpan. I excerpt from her words:

> All right, I've been putting this off ... five biopsies in eight years following up on that first diagnosis of lobular carcinoma in situ ... 'A marker of higher risk', that first breast surgeon kept repeating, and I in turn repeated it like a mantra. 'Not breast cancer, but a marker of higher risk.' He wanted to take 'em both off. No breasts, no breast cancer. I did my research, found a more conservative surgeon, and weighed the odds. Twenty to thirty per cent higher risk than the general population. At that time one woman out of every ten or eleven got breast cancer. Now it's one out of eight or nine. 'You're more likely to die in a car accident', Dr. Love had said. Since I didn't own a car, I didn't know quite what to make of that.
>
> (102–103)

Rainer understands the deadly looniness of being lumped into a statistical aggregate that does not represent your own body but that nonetheless you are told represents your probable statistical future. As she dryly puts it, '"You're more likely to die in a car accident", Dr Love had said. Since I didn't own a car, I didn't know quite what to make of that.' Rainer also knows that self-deception is one of her preferred strategies for survival. She reports having practised an ironic form of statistical thrift, shopping for lower odds, which would presumably result in a lower medical bill. It is clear that at this point she existed in the stressful ambiguous state, new to the postmodern culture of medical risk, that Sandra Gifford has so astutely identified as being 'somewhere between health and disease' (1986: 215).

While Rainer delivers these words she opens the left side of her robe to reveal her mastectomy scar. At a chance moment, we thus learn, her risk had climbed to 100 per cent. As Rainer reports later in the film, rehearsing the paradoxically improbable moment of diagnosis, 'One day I didn't have cancer and the next day I did' (1996: 17). Her upper body literally shows the outcome of some of the statistics she continues to cite throughout the film: one out of every nine women will get breast cancer. She is one of those women. But other statistics are still out there, radiating risk. In fact the odds seem to be increasing at a crazy-making rate. It is as if Rainer is living to the terrifying tempo of a statistical countdown. One out of every eight women will get breast cancer. One out of every seven. Six. In a situation such as hers statistical panic may be never-ending – until it is fatal. Five. Four. 'Thirty women die from breast cancer every hour', she reports later in the film in voice-over, 'That's one every two minutes. By the year 2000 cancer will be the leading killer of everyone' (109).

In a brilliant sequence of jump cuts, still facing the camera, Rainer tells us about the ever-present strange feeling of tightness in her skin after the mastectomy and also intones the death rates from cancer, showing us how the phenomenology of the body and statistical panic intersect in harrowing ways. I quote this passage at some length:

> I'm a sucker for statistics. They make your head spin with the dizzy-ing prospect that the body is a quantitative entity, and death can be determined with easy calculation. In the United States cancer is the leading killer of women between the ages of thirty-five and forty-five ... At first you feel a tremendous tautness across this area ... That means 2.8 million women have breast cancer ... and you have very limited mobility in your arm. Of 182,000 women newly diag-nosed with breast cancer in 1993, 46,000 will be dead in five years ... They give you exercises (*she demonstrates*) ... more than 75,000 will be dead in ten years ... and after a few months you regain almost a full range of motion. One out of nine women will develop breast cancer sometime in her life. That rate has more than doubled in the last thirty years. That taut feeling, however, never quite disap-pears. One out of three Americans will face some form of cancer. Of these, two out of three will die from the disease. That taut feeling ... The death rate ... however, never quite disappears ... from breast cancer has not been reduced in more than fifty years ... Yet there are some of us who escape ... and some of us survive.
> (*She crosses her arms and takes the 'macho' pose.*) (108)

It is as if this stutter-like sequence could go on for ever, oscillating between the palpable feeling of her body where once her breast had been and the probable prospect of death, which is the ultimate impli-cation of these disembodied statistics, figures that themselves con-stantly change at what seems to be a dizzying speed but one that can also seem boringly slow. In *MURDER and murder* statistics, both fully formed and fragmented, virtually metastasise in every direction, mate-rialising everywhere. They appear on the walls. They are written on the floor. They are posted running across the bottom of the screen like the stock market figures on a financial cable TV channel.

If the fictional woman from *Chicago Hope* reacts to her familial history of statistics with determined certitude (in that reductive narrative, she has only one conclusive figure to deal with – 86 per cent), Rainer shops for other statistics. She acts like a postmodern version of Simmel, calculating and enumerating, but she is shopping for the odds. She weighs her chances, worrying, worrying. Thus the affect of statistical panic is fundamentally related to the experience of uncertainty. Freud provides a distinction between anxiety and fear in *Inhibitions, Symptoms and Anxiety* that is useful here. Anxiety, he insists, 'has an unmistakable relation to *expectation*'; unlike fear, which is attached to a specific object, anxiety 'has a quality of *indefiniteness and lack of object*' (1926: 165). Statistical panic falls somewhere in between the two. Like anxiety, it is related to the expectation that something may happen in the future, but unlike anxiety, it is not so vague or indefinite. Yet, unlike fear – the fear, say, of being in the path of an oncoming train – statistical panic is not related to a known object that exists for us in the present. Rather it is related to a probability, to varying scenarios, to futures that are statistical in nature. When we are angry, our anger is directed at a specific object, most often a person; our anger binds us to that person. In his book on the emotions Jean-Paul Sartre, for example, draws on anger as a model for the way emotions bind us to the world. As he puts it, 'the affected subject and the affective object are bound in an indissoluble synthesis. Emotion is a certain way of apprehending the world' (1948: 52). But how can we be bound to something indefinite? To a statistic? To a figure that represents a possible future, and thus a narrative, but is at the same time a fragment of a series of possibilities? This ambiguity accounts in part for the peculiar quality of statistical stress, if not panic.

How do you live when you are at such risk? Alice Wexler provides a different answer to this question in her remarkable *Mapping Fate: A Memoir of Family, Risk, and Genetic Research*. This sensitive account contains two narratives that are as intertwined as the double helix: Wexler's personal story as the daughter of a mother who suffered from Huntington's disease, and the scientific story of the search for the gene that causes Huntington's (it was discovered in 1993). In particular, Wexler, as she writes in the introduction, is concerned to illuminate the 'emotional meanings of being at risk' for a devastating and terminal disease such as Huntington's that has no known cure (xvii). She is interested in conveying what it is like to live in its 'toxic shadow' (xix–xx). For the body inhabited by Huntington's disease is at the end a depressed body, a body that cannot communicate, a spastic body suffering from chorea or involuntary movement.

Unlike Rainer's *MURDER and murder*, *Mapping Fate* does not deluge us with statistics. But one figure of a statistical body haunts the entire narrative: 50–50. When Alice Wexler learned in 1968 (she was then in her mid-twenties) that her mother had been diagnosed with Huntington's, she simultaneously learned that she had a 50 per cent chance of inheriting the disease. Although her father told her that her immediate response to the even odds was 'That's not so bad' (43), in fact she was overpowered by this uncertain knowledge, which was transformed into denial and translated into uncertainty about her own talents for living. As her sister Nancy Wexler (a psychologist and activist for Huntington's) was later to write, 'the ambiguous condition of 50 per cent risk is extremely difficult to maintain in one's mind, if not impossible. In practice a 50–50 risk translates to a 100 per cent certainty that one will or will not develop the disease' (223). Wexler couldn't weigh the odds to determine which was heavier, as we are counselled to do as a way of solving the problem of what course of action to take, for they weighed exactly the same. Instead, her mother became a kind of mirror for her of her future body, one that she would often deny, turning away from her mother as if she were turning a mirror to the wall. 'As a feminist', she writes in the introduction, 'I particularly wanted to examine the relations between genetics and gender in our family, since I knew it somehow mattered to my own experience of growing up female that my mother – my same-sexed parent – was the parent at risk and that she was the one had developed the disease' (xvii). '*What map of the body is taken in by the daughter who sees chorea memories written on her mother's face?*' (xvii), she asks. But by the book's end she comes to feel an appreciation for her mother's grace under the pressure of the disease and thus a positive identification with her, one that allows her to dedicate *Mapping Fate*, itself a book of great clarity and honesty, to the memory of her mother.

Wexler's anxiety – her statistical panic – is palpable throughout the pages of her book as she apprehensively inspects herself for the signs of the disease, witnesses her mother's long and harrowing descent into Huntington's, offers her help in the search for the dreaded gene, and tries to get pregnant (understanding all the while the tragic future that could be in store for her child and the all-too predictable guilt she would suffer as a consequence). With a horrifying irony, the discovery of the gene and the development of a test for it, as she writes, 'opened an abyss in all our lives, a vast space between prediction and prevention' (221).

Now her anxiety about whether or not she carries the gene for Huntington's is compounded by her anguish over what might be the emotional effects of the results of the test itself. As she discovered in talking with people at risk for Huntington's in the United States, virtually 'everyone mentioned the need to escape the oppressive uncertainty' of genetic inheritance (236). They also reported that as they grew older their anxiety increased even though the odds of having the disease decrease with age. Interestingly enough, the way in which people in the United States who come from families with an incidence of Huntington's disease understand their future is culturally specific to those who live in a society saturated by the discourse of risk. As Wexler tells us, people who live in San Luis, a small community in Venezeula racked with Huntington's, have a different way of apprehending their future, of acknowledging what they are in fact certain is their inheritance. 'The people here believe that everyone who has a parent with the disease always inherits it from that parent, but only some people actually develop the symptoms', she explains. Wexler herself then assimilates their way of handling disease to our scientific category of risk, to our discourse of statistical probability. 'Perhaps it is a way', she reflects, 'of acknowledging the emotional burdens of being at risk, and the worry of constantly wondering when and if you'll get the disease. Being at risk means being different, from those who are not at risk and from those with Huntington's. It's a state all its own.' Her generous conclusion is that these people 'seem, to understand this – better, perhaps, than North Americans, who do not tolerate ambiguity well' (198–99). As she describes it, this is another instance of the new medicalisation of the body, of living in a state between health and disease.

Ultimately Wexler, having endured so long with this statistical condition, makes a kind of peace with being at risk. She chooses to reject the test for which she had thought she longed (the test, it is important to remember, does not provide absolute prediction but rather narrows the probabilities). She makes a conscious decision to choose to live in risk, refusing the cognitive map of her body that is held out to her in the form of genetic testing and statistical probabilities. She elects to face a future that holds two possibilities rather than one virtual certainty, a future that she can now name a destiny, one that for her remains open. In Wexler's *Mapping Fate* we not only see a nuanced and strong portrayal of what it feels like to be caught in the tension between the scientific language of risk and its experiential dimension. We also see how her analysis of her own statistical panic, understood as uncertainty about the future of her body, allowed her to put the paralysing implications of the number 50–50 behind her and to live into a future not ruled by a statistical roll of the dice. Thus at base, she tells us, her story is 'less about an illness than about the possibility of an illness, less about the medical dilemma of living with disease than about the existential dilemma of living at risk' (xxii). In effect Wexler redefines risk. Instead of risk ominously waiting for her in the future in the form of a statistical probability, Wexler chooses to risk fate. She decides to live in a 'third space,' one that is neither certainty nor complete uncertainty, because she has taken the action of refusing the test for the gene that causes Huntington's (xv). She takes a risk. She risks an untimely death, choosing to live, in the words of Gillian Rose, 'before her time'.[8]

III

The language of statistical probability that characterises postmodern society is a discourse in the Foucauldian sense that, like capitalism, has a history of development. In *The Taming of Chance* (1990) Hacking argues that probability is 'the philosophical success story of the first half of the twentieth century', a development he traces to the consolidation of statistical thinking in the nineteenth century, one made possible by the systematic collection of data starting around 1820, the beginning of an 'avalanche of printed numbers' that continues to deluge us today (18). By the late nineteenth century the statistical concept of the 'normal' was, according to Hacking, 'the premier statistical idea' (145), a concept that continues to have force today but has also taken, I would argue, a paradoxical turn. In the nineteenth century the normal was associated with the state of health. But if we are today everywhere and always at risk, the normal seems virtually sure to turn catastrophically into its opposite at any moment. Indeed, to be normal is to be in a state of risk, a state that at some inevitable future time will be fulfilled as a state of disease, accident, violence or death. At the turn of the twenty-first century in the society of the statistic, the sense of one's body being as risk has been internalised by virtually everyone in our consumer culture.

In this chapter, focusing on the medical body as it is represented in illness narratives, I have been interested in how contemporary cultural texts of different kinds – among them, primetime TV, experimental film and the memoir – contribute to, dissect, confront and reject the statistical body. Many other texts, of course, bear witness to the subjective experience of illness as something palpably distinct from the clinical understanding of disease as organic dysfunction.[9] And many of them also resist the lure of conflating one's own unique body with the aggregate body of statistical risk. These stories are antidotes to the often ennervating effects of the discourse of risk. If I have previously focused on texts that portray women's bodies at risk, my intent has not been to suggest that the medical statistical body is gendered female. In closing, then, I will refer briefly to one last text, *The Noonday Demon* (2001), Andrew Solomon's remarkable book on clinical depression, an illness he takes care to insist is a bodily disease. In addition to tracing the history of depression and examining the cultural politics of depression as well as its treatments, Solomon presents us with the scientific research that outlines the contours of the statistical body of clinical depression. Approximately 3 per cent of all Americans suffer from chronic depression. Nearly one in ten Americans will experience a major episode of depression in their lifetimes. Women are twice as likely to suffer depression as men. Solomon does not ignore the statistics of depression. But neither does he submit to them. It is his conviction that, as he says, 'the hard numbers are the ones that lie' (13). 'Many authors derive a rather nauseous air of invincibility from statistics', he writes, 'as though showing that something occurs 82.7 per cent of the time is more palpable and true than showing that something occurs about three out of four times' (13). Instead, the primary goal of his book is 'empathy', and with great insight and in prose that often rises to eloquence, he tells us his own harrowing story and the stories of others, conveying to us the devastating experience that is depression, one that can be 'described only in metaphor and allegory' (12, 16) and definitively not in terms of the impersonal statistical body.

Acknowledgements

I am grateful in particular to Justine Coupland, Paul Brodwin and Steven Katz for their helpful remarks as I worked on this chapter as well as to audiences at the University of Giessen in Germany, the Queensland Art Gallery in Brisbane and the University of Washington in Seattle.

Notes

1. For a more general discussion of statistics in postmodern culture, see my essay 'Statistical Panic,' from which this chapter has been adapted.
2. This figure has been disputed. In an opinion piece on the editorial page of the *New York Times* on 11 September 1997, Sally L. Satel, a psychiatrist and lecturer at the Yale School of Medicine, insists that the number is much smaller. 'Injuries from domestic assaults', she concludes, 'still accounted for just half of 1 per cent of female emergency cases in 1994.'
3. Within the domain of the market, predictability is itself a commodity; uncertainty itself has a price, one that is attached to what are called securities;

more predictability means less risk. But within the domain of our own lives the calculus of risk can produce not security but panic. On the other hand, as Edith Wyschogrod so aptly pointed out in discussion at the symposium on 'Postmodernism and the *Fin de Siècle*,' held at the University of Giessen in January 1998, there is also an erotics of risk, one that involves the desire to test oneself and to succeed against the odds, to beat the statistics, as in sports, for example, or in gambling. On the banal level of everyday life, there is the hope that we (meaning 'I') will win the lottery. There is a romance with risk, as exemplified in the popular book by Lynn Ponton entitled *The Romance of Risk*.

4. I am alluding to a short piece in the *New York Times Sunday Magazine* for 8 August 1999. Under the title 'Living Dangerously: The Odds', a list of nine different risks are taken from *Danger Ahead: The Risks You Really Face on Life's Highway*, by Larry Laudan. We learn that the odds that we will crush our finger with a hammer are one in 3000, that our doctor is really not a doctor are one in fifty, that our next meal will come from McDonald's is one in eight, and so on.

5. The counterpart of this would be statistical hope. A couple having difficulty conceiving a child and, as is said, 'given' a 3 per cent chance of succeeding, may imaginatively count themselves among that lucky 3 per cent. Similarly, many of us speak of winning the lottery, a statistical improbability of astronomical proportions (never mind an impossibility when one doesn't actually buy into the pool).

6. In January 1999 the Mayo Clinic released a study that reported on the results of what is called a bilateral prophylactic mastectomy in 639 women. It was concluded that the drastic operation reduced their chances of dying from breast cancer by 90 per cent. Out of that figure 18 women's lives were saved – but that means that 619 women had the operation performed needlessly. See Christine Gorman's 'Radical Surgery'. On 4 April 2000 the *New York Times* reported the findings from a long-term study that included women with genetic defects in the genes BRCA1 and BRCA2 resulting in the very highest risk for developing breast cancer (56 to 85 per cent); it was found that a bilateral prophylactic mastectomy reduced their risk by 90 per cent. See Denise Grady's 'Removing Healthy Breasts'.

7. That corporate America calls on the discourse of risk to sell its products – even in the instance of the prevention of disease – can be seen in the following example. On 13 November 1997 it was reported in the *New York Times* that a recent study revealed 'that cholesterol-lowering drugs could help even healthy middle-aged people with ordinary cholesterol levels reduce their risk of heart trouble by more than one-third' ('Cholesterol Drugs Shown to Cut Healthy Group's Risk,' A13). The drug, named Mavacor, costs about $100 per month. Who paid for the research? Merck and Company, the maker of the drug.

8. See Mary Russo's powerful essay on risking anachronism and the untimeliness of death where she discusses Rose's work, in particular *Love's Work: A Reckoning with Life*, in the context of ageing.

9. Gifford's distinction between these two different dimensions of risk corresponds to the medical anthropologist Arthur Kleinman's distinction between disease, represented in scientific discourse as organic dysfunction, and illness, the patient's experience of the condition.

References

Bauman, Z. (1992) 'Survival as a Social Construct', *Theory, Culture and Society* 9: 1–36.

Beck, U. 'From Industrial Society to the Risk Society: Questions of Survival, Social Structure, and Ecological Enlightenment', *Theory, Culture and Society* 9: 97–123.

— 1992 *Risk Society: Toward a New Modernity*, trans. M. Ritter. London: Sage.

Benjamin, W. (1969) 'Theses on the Philosophy of History,' *Illuminations*, ed. H. Arendt, trans. H. Zohn. New York: Schocken.

Brody, J. (2001) 'Don't Lose Sight of Real, Everyday Risks', *New York Times* 9 Oct, natl. ed: D6.

Bunton, R., Nettleton, S.N. and Burrows, R. (1995) 'Sociology and Health Promotion: Health, Risk and Consumption under Late Modernism,' Bunton, Nettleton and Burrows (eds) *The Sociology of Health Promotion: Critical Analyses of Consumption, Lifestyle and Risk*. London: Routledge, pp. 1–12.

'Cholesterol Drugs Shown to Cut Healthy Group's Risk,' *New York Times* 13 November. 1997, national edn: A13.

Freud, S. *Inhibitions, Symptoms and Anxiety* (1926), *The Standard Edition of the Complete Psychological Works of Sigmund Freud*, trans. and ed. J. Strachey, vol. 20: 77–175. London: Hogarth and Institute of Psychoanalysis, 1953–74.

Gifford, S.M. (1986) 'The Meaning of Lumps: A Case Study of the Ambiguities of Risk', C.B. Janes, R. Stall, and S.M. Gifford (eds) *Anthropology and Epidemiology: Interdisciplinary Approaches to the Study of Health and Disease* (Boston: D. Reidel, 1986), 213–46.

Gorman, C. (1999) 'Radical Surgery', *Time* 25 Jan: 83.

Grady, D. (2000) 'Removing Healthy Breasts Found Effective in High Cancer-Risk Group', *New York Times* 4 April, national edn: D7.

Hacking, I. (1990) *The Taming of Chance* (Cambridge: Cambridge University Press).

Katz, S. (1997) 'Secular Morality,' A.M. Brandt and P. Rozin *Morality and Health* (eds) New York: Routledge, 297–330.

Kleinman, A. (1988) *Illness Narratives: Suffering, Healing, and the Human Condition*. New York: Basic Books.

Lazarre, J. (1998) *Wet Earth and Dreams: A Narrative of Grief and Recovery*. Durham: Duke University Press.

'Living Dangerously: The Odds', *New York Times Sunday Magazine* 8 August 1999: 15.

'Next Frontiers', *Newsweek* 25 June 2001: 41ff.

Ponton, L.E. (1998) *The Romance of Risk: Why Teenagers Do the Things They Do* New York: Basic Books.

Rainer, Y. (1997) *MURDER and murder*. Screenplay. *Performing Arts Journal* 55: 76–117. *MURDER and murder*. Film. Dir. Y. Rainer. 113 min. Zeitgeist Films, 1996.

Rose, G. (1997) *Love's Work: A Reckoning with Life*. New York: Schocken.

Rose, P. (1997) *A Year of Reading Proust: A Memoir in Real Time*. New York: Scribner.

Russo, M. (1999) 'Aging and the Scandal of Anachronism', K. Woodward (ed.) *Figuring Age: Women, Bodies, Generations*. Bloomington: Indiana Universuty Press, 20–33.

Sartre, J.-P. (1948) *The Emotions: Outline of a Theory*, trans. B. Frechman. New York: The Philosophical Library.

Satel, S.L. (1997) 'Feminist Number Games', Editorial, *New York Times* 11 September, natl. edn.

Simmel, G. (1971) 'The Metropolis and Modern Life', 1903. trans. E.A. Shils. *On Individuality and Social Forms*. Ed. D.N. Levine. Chicago: University of Chicago Press, pp. 324–39.

Solomon, A. (2001) *The Noonday Demon: An Atlas of Depression*. New York: Scribner.

'2 People in 15 Years Killed by Turbulence', *International Herald Tribune* 30 December 1997: 4.

Wexler, A. (1995) *Mapping Fate: A Memoir of Family, Risk, and Genetic Research*. New York: Random House.

Wexler, N.S. (1979) 'Genetic "Russian Roulette": The Experience of Being "At Risk" for Huntington's Disease', S. Kessler (ed.) *Genetic Counseling: Psychological Dimensions*, New York: Academic Press.

Williams, R. (1977) 'Structures of Feeling', Williams, *Marxism and Literature*, Oxford: Oxford University Press, pp. 128–35.

Woodward, K. (1999) 'Statistical Panic', *differences* 11(2): 177–203.

Zenk, J.L. (2001) 'Advant Rx-Joint Health: An Arthritis Breakthrough', *Total Health* 23(2): 64.

12

'I am Normal on the 'Net': Disability, Computerised Communication Technologies and the Embodied Self

Deborah Lupton and Wendy Seymour

Introduction

The first part of the title of this chapter comes verbatim from a comment given in response to an on-line interview by Rita, a 56-year-old Australian living with Tourette's Syndrome, Attention Deficit Disorder and learning disorders. When asked how using computerised communication technologies had contributed to her life, she replied:

> There are so many benefits. I am constantly using my mind, eye–hand skills, meeting new people, finding relatives, keeping in touch with friends, relatives, all over the world. I can access information at any time. It is unbelievable the difference it has made to my life. I am normal on the 'Net.[1]

Rita's story is one of three case studies presented in this chapter, used to explore issues of subjectivity, embodiment and disability in relation to the use of computerised communication technologies (henceforth CCTs). These include the Internet ('Net) or World Wide Web and its associated technologies such as email, websites, bulletin boards and multi-user domains. The case studies are derived from a qualitative study that sought to understand how various new technologies, including but not limited to those used for communication, affect the experiences and subjectivities of people with disabilities.[2] Even though many people with disabilities use a range of technologies to assist their everyday functioning, surprisingly little sociocultural research exists that has sought to investigate the phenomenological and discursive aspects of this interaction.

Underpinning our notion of technology is the understanding that the term may refer to any material artefact that enhances human prowess or compensates for dysfunction. All technologies compensate in some way for aspects of embodiment that are socially and culturally perceived as limiting in certain specific contexts, whether it be a pair of spectacles, a motor vehicle, a can-opener, a spear or a personal computer. As such, all technologies, for all users, may be viewed as acting as 'prostheses' for the body. Moreover, the interaction between technologies and users is not a simple one-way process: just as users may manipulate technologies, technologies also manipulate users' bodies and subjectivities (Idhe, 1990; Latour, 1992). In many cases, as they are appropriated into everyday life, technologies may be experienced as becoming part of one's body/self: transiently or permanently.

Technologies, therefore, do not stand apart from culture, but rather are imbricated within cultural meaning. They are central to the ways in which we understand and experience our bodies and our selves. Discourse is clearly central to the interactions between technologies, bodies and selves, for it is a vehicle for conveying and reproducing the meanings that are bestowed upon technologies. Our study was generated by the quest to understand how certain technologies are used in the context of the experience of bodily limitation caused by significant physical disability, including the meanings given to this experience and the discourses employed to convey these meanings. While the research agenda consisted of a number of related questions, the question 'For people with disabilities, what discourses frame ways of understanding disability in the context of CCTs?' informs the discussion pursued in this chapter. Before discussing our case studies, in order to contextualise our research we bring together two relevant literatures: on the body and disability, and on cyberbodies.

The body and disability

A substantial literature exists in which the social and cultural meanings of disability are identified and critiqued. While the central tenet of the social model of disability (Drake, 1999: 13) is the disabling effect of social structural factors on people with impairments (Abberley, 1987; Oliver, 1996), several writers within this perspective have begun to draw upon sociological writings on the body in order to illuminate the social and cultural aspects of disabled embodiment (see, for example, Oliver, 1990; Hevey, 1992; Shakespeare, 1994; Stone, 1995; Davis, 1997; Thomson, 1997). As these writers have argued, the body with disabilities is both socially marginalised and gazed upon as a spectacle because of its cultural status as 'abnormal', 'freakish' and 'deficient'. People with disabilities are typically represented as Other, as visible evidence of the frail and constraining body and as constant reminders of mortality. They are also culturally coded as Other because of their status as marginal, liminal and anomalous in breaching notions and discourses of what is considered to be human and normal. As Robert Murphy has put it: 'The long-term physically impaired are neither sick nor well, neither dead nor alive, neither out of society nor wholly in it. They are human beings but their bodies are warped or malfunctioning, leaving their full humanity in doubt' (cited in Shakespeare, 1994: 295).

Feminist writers and those writing about race and ethnicity have been important in influencing writers on the body and disability. They share a focus on the ways in which certain types of body in specific sociocultural and historical moments are marginalised and constructed as Other. Such critics focus on the power relations underpinning cultural and social processes of identifying difference and positioning a certain type of body – typically the archetypal young, white, male, able-bodied body – as the ideal. Hughes and Paterson (1997: 332) use the term 'oppressed bodies' to refer to the types of body that are positioned as Other to this ideal. This term emphasises the interaction between power relations, discourses and Otherness in notions about 'normal' bodies as they are defined in comparison with 'abnormal' or 'deficient' bodies.

Dominant discourses are central in the Othering of bodies with disabilities. Writers in disability studies have pointed to the importance of understanding discourse as a means of giving meaning to bodily dysfunction or disability. As they argue, disability cannot be understood without reference to the culture and its realm of signification in which it is experienced and lived. Disability is not simply a physical phenomenon but also, inextricably, a sociocultural one. What is understood and accepted to be a 'disability' is always socially and culturally located and constructed via discourse. Thus, for example, there are several resonant and recurring binary oppositions in text and talk that constantly serve to position people with disabilities as Other and as deficient. These oppositions include: normal/freakish, capable/helpless, strong/weak and whole/damaged. Many disability activists seek to contest and undermine these oppositions and other powerful aspects of discourse on disabilities (see, for example, Oliver, 1990; Hevey, 1992).

Cyberbodies

In the past decade, much literature has been published on the implications of new CCTs for human subjectivity and embodiment. It is here that the concept of cyberbodies has become dominant (examples include the essays published in collections edited by Featherstone and Burrows, 1995 and Bell and Kennedy, 2000). Such literature has sought to investigate the implications for how people using CCTs experience not only social relationships but also selfhood and embodiment. Indeed, according to Bell (2000: 4), aspects of the 'human-machine interface' raise such questions as: 'Are we now so inseparable from our computers that we have effectively become them? Are they us?' Such musings go beyond the notion of CCTs as prostheses to positioning them as integral to the experience and ontology of the body/self.

The literature on the ways in which bodies/selves are mediated via CCTs tends towards a utopian representation in which bodies/selves are seen to be highly malleable. Through computerised communication, it is argued, we may become whomever we wish, we may choose to represent our bodies and selves in any way we please and even become 'posthuman' (see, for example, Haraway, 1991; Halberstam and Livingston, 1995). This is because the fleshly body is invisible on the Web: all that others know of our bodies is that information we choose to communicate to them. Men, for example, may present themselves as women, straights as gays and vice versa. Much of the literature on cyberbodies has focused on erotic exchanges on bulletin boards or chat groups, showing that participants enjoy the opportunity to take on divergent sexual identities when presenting their erotic selves to others.

Yet, while offering freedom and creative possibilities, such writings reveal a disdain or even contempt for the physicalities of the 'real body': that object which envelops ourselves. If the promise of cyberspace is that we can transmute our bodies by choosing the manner in which we represent them to others, then this implies that most of us possess bodies that constrain or limit us in some ways. Notions of normality, in turn, are implicit in these ways of thinking about the cyberbody, or the body that we construct through interactions with others via CCTs. Emphasised here is the idea of the body as performative in its malleability and capacity for the expression of multiple selves. The new CCTs 'make it much more difficult than it used to be to impose a one-to-one relationship between a single body and a single discursive identity, or . . . to warrant, to guarantee or ground, social identity in a physical body' (Foster, 2000: 445). For the utopian visions of cyberbodies appearing in some accounts, the body becomes almost entirely discursive in its release from the corporeal.

The disabled body in cyberspace

This freedom to represent the self in divergent ways, to remake the self, has been championed in both popular and academic writings on cyberculture. However, there is very little literature that deals with the ways in which people with ill or damaged bodies use the Internet. Most of the writings on embodiment in cyberculture assume that users of CCTs do not have disabilities. While they begin from the premise that the body might be transcended to some degree in cyberspace, its definitions altered and its limitations overcome, most writers in this area assume a lack of significant disability (other than the limitations that are inevitable for any fleshly body). Nor has the disability literature sought to investigate people with disabilities' interaction with CCTs to any significant extent. CCTs may offer a host of ways for people with disabilities to overcome limitations and to engage actively in social interaction in ways that were previously unavailable to them. But conversely disability can limit access to the self-transformation offered by CCTs from the very beginning: if the computer itself cannot be used because of a problem with physical co-ordination or visual impairment, or if poverty resulting from disability precludes access to a computer.

One discussion that has relevance for our research, although it is not specifically focused on disability, is Featherstone's (1995) account of the ways in which CCTs may contribute to the embodied experiences of older people (many of whom also have disabilities). He argues that the aged infirm or disabled body may often be experienced as a 'body as a prison', in which people feel trapped behind the 'mask of ageing', or the physical signs of ageing which are stigmatised in Western societies (see also Hepworth: this volume). Like the body with disabilities, the aged body is disempowered because of its sociocultural marginalisation and representation as abnormal and grotesque. Escape from this body may be sought in fantasy or daydreams, vicarious experiences via the media (especially television and film), or in the virtual reality made possible by CCTs.

As Featherstone argues, the distancing from the external realities of the body, or the opportunity to hide the 'mask of ageing', opens up new possibilities for intimacy and self-expression, including sexual expression. Some of the technologies of which he writes, such as the 'teledildonics' of interactive virtual reality sexual encounters,[3] have yet to enjoy mainstream use. But other CCTs, such as bulletin boards, multi-user domains and email, offer ways to develop intimate, and possibly erotic, relationships through verbal interactions. If CCTs offer such possibilities to the individual struggling with a marginalised ageing body, then the same may be true of people with disabilities.

Our study

The data for our study were obtained via two phases.[4] The first phase involved face-to-face semi-structured interviews with fifteen people with disabilities, carried out in 1998, about broad issues to do with their use of technologies. The nine men and six women represented a range of disabilities: paralysis as a result of spinal injuries, cerebral palsy, visual impairments and one had had a limb amputated. The second phase drew on the findings of the first to focus more specifically on disabled people's use of computerised communication technologies. Interviews with twenty people with disabilities were carried out on-line in 1999. All the research participants in the first phase lived in the Australian city of Adelaide, but those in the second phase were disbursed around Australia. The nine men and eleven women involved in the second phase again represented a wide range of disabilities, including spinal injuries, visual impairment, chronic fatigue syndrome, hearing impairment, cerebral palsy, acquired brain injury, Tourette's syndrome, multiple sclerosis and arthritis (some of the participants were living with more than one of these disabilities). Nearly all of the participants were aged between 30 and 60, with none older than this and only two aged in their twenties.

Our decision to use on-line interviewing for the second phase was based on several key principles that underpinned the research. First, our overriding intention was to create a research context that encouraged easy participation and enabled the participants to influence the direction of the research. Second, we were investigating on-line practices: the integrity of the research demanded that we employ on-line interviews.

Participants were recruited by electronic means using a readily available list server with a wide circulation. A clear statement in the initial project information described the mechanics and rationale of the selection process and ensured that the volunteers were aware of the dimensions of the research and the time that they might need to commit to the project. While the recruitment process presupposed a certain degree of computer expertise, the conduct of the research explicitly sought to diminish the effects of any 'mystique of methods' (Mann and Stewart, 2000: 29) into the process of the research. A threaded[5] on-line discussion site provided by the university at which one of us was employed allowed us to post open-ended interview questions which participants could answer at any time, including re-entering the site later to complete answers. We were able to read previous replies as they were sent, and to ask further questions based on these replies, resulting in a semi-structured interview format. We found that this method of data collection was very fruitful, with many participants giving long and thoughtful replies to our questions, obviously taking time to consider them before replying (an opportunity which is less available in the more spontaneous spoken interview format). Freeing data collection from the constraints of the visible body, location and time are significant elements in liberating the interview from the constraints of traditional face-to-face qualitative research. The interview is more open, more discursive, less pre-constructed and less dominated by the corporeal presence of either researcher or participant (Seymour, 2001).

Because of the self-selected nature of the research participants, the data we collected are not generalisable to the wider population of people with disabilities. There are many disabilities that were not represented among the participants and, by its very nature, those people who are unable to access personal computers and the Internet would not have been able to be included in the second phase of our study. Despite its limitations, however, our data provided us with some rich insights into the ways in which some people with disabilities use CCTs and other technologies.

The data from the first phase of our study revealed the high importance that people with disabilities attached to computerised technologies, particularly those used for communication (see Lupton and Seymour, 2000). All the participants used CCTs, and many said that they relied upon them to function each day. The most commonly used of such technologies were personal computers (some of which were voice-activated or talking computers), electronic organisers or memo machines and scanners. The majority of participants used personal computers for wordprocessing and for communication purposes via email and bulletin boards.

When discussing the attributes of the technologies they used, communication with others emerged as one of the most important, as did autonomy, control over one's body and life, independence, competence, confidence, the ability to engage in the workforce and the opportunity to participate as part of the wider community. For example, those participants who said that they used interactive bulletin boards noted that this allowed them to share experiences, ideas and resources with others also sharing their disability. Such technologies, therefore, were important in contributing to participants' knowledge of their disability and giving them emotional and practical support when it was required. This avenue of communication was important for their identity as part of a group of people with particular disabilities. Another important theme of the interviews, however, was the participants' insistence that their self-identity not be solely defined by their disability. According to those who used them, it was here that CCTs came into their own. They saw such technologies as facilitating communication because they had a choice about whether or not to reveal their disability to others. As such, these participants felt that they were able to avoid the discrimination, stigmatisation and patronising attitudes that they had experienced in other communication contexts. In the second phase of the study, it was clear that these themes required further exploration. We chose three case studies from among the twenty people we interviewed. These case studies were chosen because of the richness of data they offered in terms of insights into the experiences of people with disabilities using CCTs and the ways they represented their bodies in discussing these experiences. Coincidentally all three people described in the case studies are women, but they each have very different types of disability. All face challenges, however, in communicating with others face-to-face because of such aspects of their embodiment as limited mobility, bodily features which render them self-conscious, an adverse reaction to the chemicals used by others or in the environment, or sheer fatigue, pain or illness. It is in this context of difficulty with interpersonal communication that Rita, Alison and Rhonda discuss their use of CCTs.

The case studies

Rita

Rita is in her fifties and lives with Tourette's Syndrome (which causes uncontrollable twitches and tics), Attention Deficit Disorder and learning difficulties. She had been using a personal computer for about six months at the time of the interview. Rita mainly uses the computer as part of her voluntary work as a disability advocate, but also to contact relatives and friends via email and the Internet. She takes part in specific disability chat sessions as part of her support work for organisations for people with Tourette's Syndrome and learning disabilities, and also participates in a general disability advocacy group. She is self-taught, and said that as a result she still lacks confidence in using the technologies.

At the time of the interview, Rita was using the computer for about an hour each day. She commented that she found learning how to operate the computer an initial barrier because of her history of learning disorders, which has undermined her confidence in tackling a learning task: 'Anything to do with learning and education has bad associations for me.' Rita also noted that when she is off her medication she finds eye–hand co-ordination and concentration very difficult, which meant that using the computer was difficult. She described her first experience of engaging in a computerised discussion group as 'a disaster' because of a lack of co-ordination associated with her disability:

> I couldn't coordinate myself quickly enough and I PANICKED. I have problems with eye-hand hand coordination – more so when I am excited and concentrating. I went into a blind panic, and still do sometimes. The first one I did was with a LD [learning disorder] chatline for adults, where I was asked to talk about how I handle my problems with dyscalculia. Numbers don't make sense to me, so I have devised a method to deal with that problem. I knew what to say – I had rehearsed it, I had my notes, then couldn't get my hands and eyes to work together, just couldn't find the letters on the keyboard. The more I tried to calm down, [the more] I dithered.

In this account of her disability, Rita represented her body as failing to deal with the demands of this particular CCT. Her body's slowness and lack of co-ordination, combined with an emotional response to this ('blind panic'), acted as a powerful disincentive to using the CCT. Rita said that she still did not really enjoy taking part in real-time discussions, because she felt that she could not respond quickly enough and as a result felt 'pressured'. However, she felt strongly motivated to continue with taking part in the chat sessions because of her desire to help others and to be a strong advocate for those with her disorders. Using the Internet, she said, was much easier and saved her time and money in communicating with other disability advocates around Australia and overseas. As such, this technology allowed her much more opportunity to make friends and feel as if she were part of a community, helping her to 'come to terms with my disability'.

Rita also discussed the way in which the computer allows her to forget her status as a 'disabled person' because she can hide aspects of her body that set her apart as different. She is extremely self-conscious about her Tourette's tics, which she is unable to control and have extremely negative social repercussions, marking her out as 'different' and 'strange':

> For me [using the computer] is great, as I am very conscious of my disability. The facial tics and body tics can be quite bad some days, 'specially when I am off medication for a while. It is comforting to know they cannot see me. And I know it is wrong, but it does make me feel safe and normal. Also I feel we are joined by a common bond that overrides the disability feature. For me, it is freedom of having to deal with someone on my bad days, yet they cannot see my tics and judge me or look at me in a way that unsettles me. I am very conscious of how others see my disability and my behaviour. Off medication I am very impulsive and talk louder and my tics are bad, although I do not have the very bad tics of the disorder.

In this excerpt, Rita's account of the implications of her disabilities underline her Otherness to others. Her words reveal her acknowledgement that her tics position her as unsettling to others. It is 'comforting' not to have to deal with the embarrassment engendered in her face-to-face interactions with others. Alone in her house, communicating via CCTs, no one with whom she communicates need know of her disabilities. This offers an anonymity which is freeing because it means she can communicate even on her 'bad days', when her body is less controllable than usual. She feels that she can escape others' judgement and can be united by a 'common bond' that would not be possible in face-to-face interaction.

Rita elaborated on how using the computer makes her 'feel normal'. She noted that she can communicate without having to control her body to make her more socially acceptable, and this for her is a great relief and freedom:

> I survived and worked within the real world hiding my disability with extremely harsh medications. Sometimes I felt I had a split personality, as the real world rarely saw me on my bad days or off medication. I never then nor still feel confident and safe enough to

go out without medication. On the 'Net, I can communicate with both normal and disabled freely and openly even when my tics are out of control. As I am typing this my head and eye tics along with my left arms and feet are twisting and jerking as I type, yet I do not have to worry about it, just concentrate on what I am doing. When I communicate with others, I am free, normal for me and totally at peace with my skin. It's heady, like I imagine what being drunk could feel like. I am also not guarded in my communication, nor do I have to waste energy watching body language and imagining how people are really responding to me, as I tried so hard to be normal. I know I am much more relaxed and at peace with myself on line.

For Rita, therefore, using a computer for communication offers a means to escape her stigmatised and stigmatising body. The sheer effort of trying to control her body can be relinquished and she can still be active in social interactions. The excerpts also reveal, however, Rita's knowledge that admitting to wanting to be 'normal' – and indeed, even using that word – counters a dominant trend in disability advocacy (with which she aligns herself in her voluntary work) to challenge the binary opposition that positions them as 'abnormal' ('I know it is wrong, but it does make me feel safe and normal'). She struggles, then, between relishing the freedom from her disabilities that CCTs offer her, and realising that such transitory freedom does not allow her to escape from the more pervasive discourses that construct her as Other in wider society, where her body betrays her. This is underlined by her reference to herself as having a 'split personality', in which her bodily problems were contained using powerful drugs, but not removed, so that the 'real' disabled self was only covered over and 'normality' illusory. So, too, the CCTs Rita uses allow her only to 'hide' her disability, and the persona she presents on-line is not the one known to the 'real world'. Nonetheless, the sheer pleasure offered by engaging in social interaction without the constraints of her body is enough to make Rita feel 'much more relaxed and at peace with myself'. Her representation of her on-line self, therefore, presents a more 'real self' that more closely approximates the 'normality' expected by others and longed for by Rita. Her body and its 'twisting and jerking' becomes irrelevant to her attempts to communicate. At the same time, she is still painfully aware that this more 'peaceful' and 'normal for me' body/self only exists for as long as she is on-line.

Alison

Alison, aged in her forties, suffered permanent physical damage when she broke her back and legs in an accident, and also suffered some brain damage. She is mobile, but has limited movement in one hand (which is wired open), endures chronic pain from her damaged spine and suffers from dizziness, lack of co-ordination and balance, and short-term memory loss. These physical problems have meant that she has difficulties moving around and travelling, and she must plan very carefully when making expeditions. As she explained in her interview:

> There are a multitude of things I have great difficulty doing. I can't bend down to pick something up, at home I use a 'pick up stick'. When I am out, I usually ask someone else to pick it up for me, or keep walking, and most of the time people pick it up and tell me I have dropped something. There are so many things I either can't do, or have great difficulty doing them. I just try very hard to organise myself so that I rarely get myself into the position of 'exposing' myself . . . I can't use public transport, I forget where I am going a lot of the time, forget where I have to get off, fall over a lot if I can't get a seat, because of my balance.

Like Rita, Alison's account of her body's failings emphasises her desire to avoid social embarrassment and being made to feel 'different' or 'deficient' in public places. Attempting to avoid 'exposure' as a person with disabilities consumes a huge amount of her effort and time. Her use of the word 'exposing' emphasises her pervasive sense that the body/self she presents in public only thinly hides the true nature and extent of her disabilities. Like Rita's accounts of her 'split personality', Alison's choice of words suggests that she feels a schism between the body/self that she presents as 'normal' to others, and the 'real' body/self that must be tightly controlled to achieve this public persona.

Alison uses her personal computer extensively, to assist her in her everyday activities (a diary that reminds her when to do things), for on-line university studies and for leisure and social interaction. She engages in interactive games (backgammon) and reads international newspapers on the Internet. She also spends an average of three hours a day chatting on the Internet to her friends, of which she has made many throughout the world by engaging in chatlines. She is very positive about this aspect of her Internet use:

I have been able to meet interesting and wonderful people who I would never have met without the Internet . . . The great thing is I can chat when I want to, or send emails when I feel like writing. There is no 'I have to reply right now' if I don't feel like it then. I can always reply at my own leisure, maybe 2 am my time (have trouble sleeping), and I know I am not waking anyone, or spending large amounts of money in phone calls.

Alison is explicit about the ways in which CCTs have allowed her to have a social life in spite of the constraints imposed upon her by her body:

Life has changed very much. For a long time I would not go out, did not try to meet friends, and with the Internet I have experienced a real change. The computer was instrumental in my initial recovery. Playing games and trying to write letters (before real wordprocessors were around) was very difficult, but I persevered, it HAD to get better, I would not accept that was it. So I just plugged on and on, now I have regular outings with friends who have ABI [acquired brain injury], and attend group meetings, Management Committee meetings, do 'talks' for government departments and anyone interested. I still love staying at home, for reasons that I am simply very happy doing so. I am not alone any more, I can come on line and either chat with a friend, or write an email, after that I can surf the 'Net to my heart's desire. Quite simply – I love it!.

Like Rita, Alison noted that using CCTs makes her feel as if she need not hide aspects of her damaged body. This makes her feel as if she can be more honest and deal with her physical problems better without fear of embarrassment:

[On the 'Net] I find it easier to just say, 'I am tired and have to go', [but] when I am speaking face to face, I find this very difficult. And when I am feeling not too well, I can simply go off-line and take myself to bed – I can't do this any other way. I don't have to get 'dressed up' to chat and do things on line as I do in person. It does not tire me as much as face-to-face communication, I don't have to worry about body language, or giving reflecting listening, I can be more objective on line . . . I love the fact that I can sit at my computer looking like something dragged from a scary film, in daggy [unfashionable] track suit, hair a mess, and drinking tea almost non stop.

As her account suggests, Alison finds it difficult to engage in face-to-face interactions because of her propensity for experiencing fatigue and pain and her belief that she must observe the social niceties. While she places less emphasis on the desire to achieve 'normality' than Rita does, and does not overtly use the word 'freedom' when describing the benefits of on-line communication, Alison's account demonstrates her pleasure at not having to force herself to present her body in ways that are socially demanded in face-to-face interaction. For Alison, it is her ability to use time as she wants that emerges as particularly freeing. She can communicate when she feels able to, at any time, including the middle of the night, and can equally conclude her interactions at any time, if she is feeling tired or unwell.

Rhonda

Rhonda, aged in her fifties, has chronic fatigue syndrome (CFS), fibromyalgia and multiple chemical sensitivity (MCS). In her interview she described how her illnesses affected her physically and mentally:

> They cause fatigue beyond the normal level – e.g. exercise causes fatigue in muscles so then one is forced to rest. There are lousy aches and pains in muscles and joints. The MCS makes it difficult in as much as I cannot be around people who are wearing perfume, for instance, as it causes nausea and bad headaches. Of course it is not simply perfumes – any sort of chemical smells – e.g. carpets and paint. One of the worst bits of these illnesses is the fact that it somehow affects the brain and we get what we call brain 'fog'. So there are times when we are unable to function the way we really want to. Can't find the words etc. Difficult with study, I can tell you. The pain etc. is worse in winter of course, and is pretty much a 24 hour thing. Affects sleep and getting about: e.g. Sat. and Sun. get papers delivered, have to use walking stick to hobble out to get them, then try valiantly to pick them up. Affects all joints. Headaches and various other symptoms such as being off balance most of time. Too many to really put in. Have a 'bad' back and hips – caused by accidents and old age. Arthritis in knees is part of ageing too.

Rhonda also found it difficult to interact physically with others because of her MCS, as perfume, for example, affected her, and many environments are full of chemicals to which she reacts badly. Like the other women described here, Rhonda was very positive about the ways in which CCTs allowed her to escape loneliness and engage in social contact with others. She said of her use of email that: 'Disability causes aloneness at times and contact with others in any form helps that and the pain and frustration.' Via CCTs she has made several friends with CFS who have provided her with emotional support.

Rhonda said that she used her computer every second day or so and used email to keep in touch with friends. She found the pace of communication on email an advantage over telephone conversations: 'When I speak via the phone, the brain may not be in gear at that time, and stress and nervousness can bring "it" [her loss of brain function] on, so this method gives me the extra time to think and work out the answers etc., and I don't get the stress.' Communication by email, therefore, allows Rhonda to overcome the stress she feels in face-to-face or real-time electronic communication engendered by her inability on some occasions to think quickly. It allows her to communicate on her own terms and at her own pace.

Although Rhonda said that she enjoyed using email, she also commented that her mental disabilities made it difficult at times. She does not use chat or discussion groups because, like Rita, she has trouble keeping up with the pace of the discussion, and finds that even to answer an email she has to print it out first and take her time responding. Rhonda's physical disabilities also made using a computer difficult in several ways. She commented that she found typing easier on an electronic keyboard than on a typewriter as she suffers joint pain in her hands, and she saw being able easily to print out documents a boon. On the other hand, she found it difficult to type at all: 'My only difficulty in email "talk" is the actual typing. When the pain and stiffness are so bad, it may take more than one episode of actual typing to get one letter done.' She went on to detail how aspects of the computer cause physical and cognitive problems, especially real-time discussion groups:

> My ability to handle so many things – and everything at a fast pace – is not good. If you were to stand in front of me and do an action with your arms, then ask me to mimic you, it would take time for my brain and body to get their acts together, and for me to actually copy you. Imagine then how my brain reacts to all these little things popping up on a screen in front of me!!!!!!!! . . . I did get very dizzy and nauseous from watching the split screen, especially when it became 3 then 4 people talking. Will give it another go, and then maybe, very unsure – occasionally. I prefer things where I can write

at my own pace, and send it off later. I can stop and go for a walk outside, or just think, or watch TV then come back when I, and my poor old brain are ready.

Rhonda's account here underlines the difficulties that some people may face when using CCTs. The technologies are designed for able-bodied people, who expect to interact with other able-bodied people when communicating via CCTs. Keeping up the pace may be very hard work for those who have some types of disability. For Rhonda, therefore, while some aspects of CCTs allow her to transcend her bodily limitations, such as her ability to have social encounters with others easily and without the risk of triggering her MCS, other features of CCTs only exacerbate or emphasise them. Unlike Rita and Alison, Rhonda is unable to experience an on-line body/self that is free, if only fleetingly, from disability. Her account, therefore, is less laudatory of CCTs than are those of the other women. For the same reasons, Rhonda speaks little of being able to hide her disabilities from others via CCTs and nor does she portray a different type of body/self constructed through CCTs that is able to escape the realities of disability.

Conclusion

Despite the politics of difference articulated by many critics within disability studies, our research suggests that 'normality', as it is defined by dominant discourses related to able-bodied interaction, is a goal that many people with disabilities seek. The body of a person with disabilities in many social realms is profoundly coded with the discourses of embodiment: being a body rather than having a body. In face-to-face communication, rather than possessing an 'absent body', a body that recedes from consciousness while the mind/self is allowed to take over (Leder, 1990), the person with a disabled body must cope with a body that is conspicuous and ever-present, at least to others. Because of this prominence and the focus that is constantly given to disability and its accoutrements such as a wheelchair or a cane, the body assumes a dominant status as an emblem of the self. Many people with disabilities complain that the visibility of their disability defines them to others, obscuring or eliminating consideration of other aspects of the self/body (see, for example, Shildrick and Price, 1996; Lupton and Seymour, 2000). While their bodies are constantly communicating to others, the meanings they communicate are themselves disabling. Their bodies 'speak' in ways that enable them to be misunderstood or misinterpreted by others, leading to stigmatisation, prejudice and discriminatory practices.

As we noted earlier in this chapter, Featherstone has used the phrase the 'mask of ageing' to capture the stigmatising nature of ageing as well as the feeling that the 'real self' – in that case, the self that is felt to be still youthful and conforming to notions of youthful attractiveness and vitality – is being hidden behind the fleshly body. Equally, the phrase the 'mask of disability' might be used to convey the feelings of our participants that their 'real selves' are neglected or ignored because of the outward bodily display of their disabilities.

Our participants wished to see themselves as 'normal', not 'abnormal', 'freakish' or 'Other'. Many people with disabilities see the 'bodylessness' of communicating via CCTs as holding a seductive promise of 'normality', or at least a route to escape from the constraints imposed by disabling discourses. It is clear that CCTs present a significant means to subvert the impact of the conspicuous body, to counter 'Otherness' and to obscure the detrimental consequences of 'differentness' on everyday social participation. In contrast to the dominant role of the body in face-to-face encounters, computer competence enables people with disabilities to take control of the interaction that transpires. Being able to communicate via CCTs means that aspects of their 'real selves' could be expressed and appreciated without the encumbering physicality of their bodies, weighed down as they are with the negative sociocultural meanings that are bestowed upon disability and difference. Their bodies, at least for a time, may be silenced, no longer 'speaking' their difference. For at least two of the women in our case studies, this allowed the emergence of an *alter ego* they considered to be liberating and more expressive of their 'true self' than was the self that was defined by the limits of their physicality.

However, the discourses of liberation and disembodiment are accompanied by accounts that 'bring the body back in' in a number of different ways. The body not only predominates as the general topic of on-line conversations for many of our interviewees, particularly on chat groups related to their disabilities, but the focus is directed to bodily imperfections, deficits and abnormalities – topics that define the body as deviant rather than 'normal'. Further, all bodies continue to make fleshly demands, even in cyberspace or virtual reality (Lupton, 1995). People with disabilities may find that the materiality of their bodies, coupled with specific aspects of their disabilities, will continue to limit the nature or scope of their interactions. The body may not move fast enough for some interactions, or may easily tire or suffer discomfort or pain while at the keyboard. People with disabilities who achieve a sense of normality when communicating with others via CCTs still must face pain, penury, discrimination and struggles to communicate and their 'true self' recognised when they log out. In this respect, the sheer corporeality of their bodies dominates over discourses of freedom and normality. The physical body may be invisible to others, but it remains a conspicuous part of the self: a phantom behind the text.

Our research, therefore, is vivid evidence of the way in which the body cannot disappear or be fully transmuted via discourse, despite the 'body-free' discourses typical of cyberculture utopias. While the body can never be free of discourse – that is, we cannot experience embodiment except through the discourses in which we are acculturated from birth – nor is discourse ever free of the body. The cultural meanings of disability do affect how we speak, think about and experience the body, including our ideas of 'normality'. But disabled embodiment is also a material reality that may affect the extent to which people may participate in the sharing of or the struggle against dominant discourses.

Notes

1. All extracts from the on-line interviews used as data in this chapter have been reproduced exactly as they were originally typed in by the participants except for the correction of spelling or typographical errors.
2. In recent writings on disability there has been a tendency for proponents of the social model of disability to make a distinction between 'impairment' and 'disability'. These writers see disability as being a social response to impairment on the part of those who are non-disabled, such that those who have some impairment are discriminated against and not provided with the appropriate facilities to allow them to function as active citizens. Impairment, therefore, is seen as the bodily phenomenon from which disability springs as the social outcome. Some critics have seen this distinction as disavowing the lived experience of disability by refusing to acknowledge the material reality that is part of living with a disability. They have also argued that the body itself (and thus impairment) can never be experienced and understood independently of sociocultural frameworks, and that to therefore draw a distinction between 'biological' impairment and 'social' disability is misguided (see, for example, Shildrick and Price, 1996; Hughes and Paterson, 1997). We have chosen here to use the term 'people with disabilities'.
3. 'Teledildonics' is a type of sexual activity using virtual reality devices attached to one's fleshly body to engage in tactile activities involving actual stimulation of erotic zones as well as audio and visual cues. Individuals using these devices may interact solely with simulated partners or with other people using the equipment.

4. This research was funded by the University of South Australia. We are grateful for this funding and to the participants in the study.
5. The threaded interview format enables 'asynchronous' on-line discussion to take place via the Internet between interviewer and interviewee. This format is distinct from the synchronous style of discussion that takes place within on-line, real-time chat groups. In contrast, the threaded interview enables both interviewer and interviewee to respond to posted messages with a dedicated private interview space at their own convenience. The posted messages are therefore maintained on the interview website in a hierarchical fashion, enabling both interviewer and interviewee to revisit previous postings across the time-span of the interview.

References

Abberley, P. (1987) 'The Concept of Oppression and the Development of a Social Theory of Disability', *Disability, Handicap & Society* 2(1): 5–19.

Bell, D. (2000) 'Introduction I: Cybercultures Reader: A User's Guide', in D. Bell and B. Kennedy (eds) *The Cybercultures Reader*. London: Routledge, pp. 1–12.

Bell, D. and Kennedy, B. (eds), (2000) *The Cybercultures Reader*. London: Routledge.

Davis, L. (1997) 'Introduction: The Need for Disability Studies', in L. Davis (ed.) *The Disability Studies Reader*. New York: Routledge. pp. 1–8.

Drake, R. (1999) *Understanding Disability Policies*. London: Macmillan.

Featherstone, M. (1995) 'Post-bodies, Aging and Virtual Reality', in M. Featherstone and A. Wernick (eds) *Images of Aging: Cultural Representations of Later Life*. London: Routledge, pp. 227–44.

Featherstone, M. and Burrows, R. (eds) (1995) *Cyberspace, Cyberbodies, Cyberpunk: Cultures of Technological Embodiment*. London: Sage.

Foster, T. (2000) 'Trapped by the Body?' Telepresence Technologies and Transgendered Performance in Feminist and Lesbian Rewritings of Cyberpunk Fiction', in D. Bell and B. Kennedy (eds) *The Cybercultures Reader*. London: Routledge, pp. 439–59.

Halberstam, J. and Livingston, I. (1995) *Posthuman Bodies*. Bloomington, IN: Indiana University Press.

Haraway, D. (1991) *Simians, Cyborgs and Women: The Reinvention of Nature*. New York: Routledge.

Hevey, D. (1992) *The Creatures Time Forgot: Photography and Disability Imagery*. London: Routledge.

Hughes, B. and Paterson, K. (1997) 'The Social Model of Disability and the Disappearing Body: Towards a Sociology of Impairment', *Disability & Society* 12(3): 325–40.

Ihde, D. (1990) *Technology and the Lifeworld*. Bloomington, IN: Indiana University Press.

Latour, B. (1992) 'Where are the Missing Masses? The Sociology of a Few Mundane Artifacts'. In W. Bijker and J. Law (eds) *Shaping Technology/Building Society: Studies in Sociotechnical Change*. Cambridge, MA. The MIT Press, pp. 225–58.

Leder, D. (1990) *The Absent Body*. Chicago: University of Chicago Press.

Lupton, D. (1995) 'The Embodied Computer/User', *Body & Society* 1(3–4): 97–112.

Lupton, D. and Seymour, W. (2000) 'Technology, Selfhood and Physical Disability'. *Social Science & Medicine* 50: 1851–62.

Mann, C. and Stewart, F. (2000) *Internet Communication and Qualitative Research: A Handbook for Researching Online*. London: Sage.

Oliver, M. (1990) *The Politics of Disablement*. London: Macmillan.

Oliver, M. (1996) *Understanding Disability: From Theory to Practice*. London: Macmillan.

Seymour, W. (2001) 'In the Flesh or Online? Exploring Qualitative Research Methodologies'. *Qualitative Research* 1(2): 147–68.

Shakespeare, T. (1994) 'Cultural Representation of Disabled People: Dustbins for Disavowal?'. *Disability & Society*, 9(3): 283–99.

Shildrick, M. and Price, J. (1996) 'Breaking the Boundaries of the Broken Body' *Body & Society*, 2(4): 93–113.

Stone, S. (1995) 'The Myth of Bodily Perfection'. *Disability & Society* 10(4): 413–24.

Thomson, R. (1997) *Extraordinary Bodies: Figuring Physical Disability in American Culture and Literature*. New York: Columbia University Press.

Index of Names

Index of Subjects